The Arnold and Caroline Rose Monograph Series
of the American Sociological Association

Religion and fertility

Arab Christian–Muslim differentials

Other books in the series

J. Milton Yinger, Kiyoshi Ikeda, Frank Laycock, and Stephen J. Cutler: *Middle Start: An Experiment in the Educational Enrichment of Young Adolescents*

James A. Geschwender: *Class, Race, and Worker Insurgency: The League of Revolutionary Black Workers*

Paul Ritterband: *Education, Employment, and Migration: Israel in Comparative Perspective*

John Low-Beer: *Protest and Participation: The New Working Class in Italy*

Orrin E. Klapp: *Opening and Closing: Strategies of Information Adaptation in Society*

Rita James Simon: *Continuity and Change: A Study of Two Ethnic Communities in Israel*

Marshall B. Clinard: *Cities with Little Crime: The Case of Switzerland*

Steven T. Bossert: *Tasks and Social Relationships in Classrooms: A Study of Instructional Organization and Its Consequences*

Richard E. Johnson: *Juvenile Delinquency and Its Origins: An Integrated Theoretical Approach*

David R. Heise: *Understanding Events: Affect and the Construction of Social Action*

Ida Harper Simpson: *From Student to Nurse: A Longitudinal Study of Socialization*

Stephen P. Turner: *Sociological Explanation as Translation*

Janet W. Salaff: *Working Daughters of Hong Kong: Filial Piety or Power in the Family?*

Religion and fertility

Arab Christian–Muslim differentials

Joseph Chamie

Cambridge University Press

Cambridge

London New York New Rochelle

Melbourne Sydney

Published by the Press Syndicate of the University of Cambridge
The Pitt Building, Trumpington Street, Cambridge CB2 1RP
32 East 57th Street, New York, NY 10022, USA
296 Beaconsfield Parade, Middle Park, Melbourne 3206, Australia

First published 1981

Printed in the United States of America
Typeset by Jay's Publishers Services, Inc., North Scituate, Mass.
Printed and bound by The Murray Printing Co., Westford, Mass.

Library of Congress Cataloging in Publication Data

Chamie, Joseph.

Religion and fertility.

(The Arnold and Caroline Rose monograph series in sociology)

Summary in Arabic.

Includes bibliographical references.

1. Fertility, Human – Lebanon – Moral and religious aspects. 2. Lebanon – Population. I. Title.
II. Series: Arnold and Caroline Rose monograph series in sociology.
HQ663.9.C47 261.8'3663 80-19787
ISBN 0 521 23677 0 hard covers
ISBN 0 521 28147 4 paperback

Contents

Tables and figures

Tables

Figures

Foreword

Our knowledge of important social-demographic interrelations is being greatly advanced by social surveys such as the study on which this book is based. Large parts of the world's population live in countries in which vital statistics and census data are grossly inadequate. New methods for utilizing such defective data to make indirect demographic estimates alleviate this situation in many cases. However, well-conducted surveys have the advantage of providing data on characteristics often not available in official statistics: religion, income, family planning, and fertility preferences in relation to actual fertility. The World Fertility Survey is providing such data for many countries of the world. However, the tragedy of the Lebanese civil war made the participation of Lebanon in this international survey impossible. It was, therefore, fortunate that the 1971 National Fertility and Family Planning Survey of Lebanon was conducted before the civil conflict and that Dr. Chamie was invited to analyze it while this was still possible.

Lebanon's demographic situation has a scientific and practical importance far greater than might be supposed from the country's relatively small population. This is a society that is a kind of social laboratory in the sense that in it one can observe important religious communities at different stages of social and economic development. It is possible in this setting to analyze the interacting effects of religion and socioeconomic development on reproductive behavior. Such an analysis is the core of this book.

Empirical analyses often contradict the simple generalizations that are made in the absence of data. For example, presumed religious differences in reproductive behavior are often deduced from theological dicta and literature. Dr. Chamie demonstrates that in Lebanon the actual attitudes and behavior with respect to fertility and contraception do not correspond to doctrinal differences.

Dr. Chamie also shows that such broad religious classifications as Christian and Muslim can be very misleading. He demonstrates, for example, that two Muslim sects have such dissimilar reproductive patterns that one resembles Christian sects, whereas the other is quite different. In view of contemporary political events, it is significant that one of these Muslim groups is Shi'a and the other is Sunni. Western observers are learning that it is important to understand the difference between Shi'a and Sunni Muslims. This is not the first time that groups that are different demographically have been found to be politically different, too.

Received wisdom is also contradicted by the interesting finding that the newest, most modern, and most effective contraceptives are used most by groups in the population that have most recently come to fertility control, that have had the highest fertility, and that are least advanced in terms of such criteria as educational level. It is interesting that the religious groups in Lebanon with the closest ties to European culture have relied most on coitus interruptus, the principal contraceptive method in the historic decline of Western European fertility. Here again, there is evidence that fertility can be brought to relatively low levels without highly sophisticated modern contraceptives, if motivation is strong enough.

Another way of putting this is that sophisticated populations can control fertility levels with what appear to be unsophisticated methods. A contemporary example on a national scale is Japan, which has maintained low fertility at replacement levels for more than twenty years by relying almost entirely on the use of the condom, with legal abortion as a backup in case of failure.[1] Recent research in Indonesia also indicates that, as in Lebanon, advanced strata of the population that have practiced contraception longest are most likely to use traditional methods rather than sophisticated modern methods.[2] In Indonesia, as in Lebanon, population strata that have more recently begun to use contraception rely largely on the modern methods.

Perhaps the most interesting theoretical issue in this book is Dr. Chamie's argument that religion and socioeconomic status interact in their effect on fertility. He shows that effects are not simply additive. Instead, it appears that religious differences are greatest for the less advanced social strata and are of much less consequence for advanced social strata. One important implication of these findings is that religious fertility differentials cannot be explained simply by the socioeconomic characteristics of the religious groups. This is consistent with cumulating evidence that customary socioeconomic characteristics appear to be insufficient to explain fertility trends and differentials without taking into account such cultural characteristics as religion, ethnicity, language, and local regional traits.

These introductory remarks have been intended to indicate that, apart from its significance for understanding Lebanon, Dr. Chamie's interesting analyses are relevant to important general issues in the comparative study of fertility.

Population Studies Center
University of Michigan

Ronald Freedman

Preface

During my involvement in this research, Lebanon was plagued with the most devastating civil conflict in its history. In the twenty-month period from April 1975 to November 1976, roughly 2 percent of the resident population in Lebanon was killed and 5 percent was injured. Without a doubt, this conflict was one of the bloodiest civil wars of the twentieth century; rarely have such high percentages of a nation's population been killed and wounded in so few months.

The research described herein is in no way intended to contribute to the divisions that are currently separating the Lebanese communities. The focuses of this investigation are both the differences and the similarities in fertility, family size preference, and family planning behavior among Lebanese religious groups. It is the author's firm belief that the recognition of such differences and similarities is more conducive to intersectarian tolerance, understanding, and cooperation than is the disregarding or denial of them. It is hoped that these results will contribute to a diminution of the divisions among the Lebanese people.

The data reported in this investigation were kindly made available to me by the Lebanon Family Planning Association. I would like to thank all the members of the association – especially their previous president, Dr. Edna Aboujdiid – for their assistance and cooperation.

My deepest thanks also go to Dr. Adnan Mroueh, Professor of Obstetrics and Gynecology at the American University of Beirut, and Dr. Louis Verhoestraete, former director of the School of Public Health of the American University of Beirut. Dr. Mroueh's guidance, encouragement, and friendship were, and continue to be, greatly appreciated. The assistance, hospitality, and all-around goodwill of Dr. Verhoestraete made my stay and work in Lebanon possible and enjoyable.

The Rockefeller-Ford Foundation's Research Program on Population and Developmental Policy provided a good part of the financial support for this investigation. I would also like to thank those at the

Rockefeller Foundation who assisted in the administration of the research grant.

The Population Studies Center of the University of Michigan provided me with an ideal environment in which to work. I am grateful to the directors, faculty, staff, and students for their support and assistance. Very special thanks are due to Professor Ronald Freedman, who in innumerable ways has been a great help to me. In addition, the comments and suggestions of Professor Albert Hermalin have added greatly to this work. I am also indebted to Professor Jason Finkle, not only for being instrumental in making it possible for us to work in Lebanon, but also for his longtime support, encouragement, and friendship. I would also like to thank all the reviewers and the editors and staff of the Cambridge University Press who so generously offered suggestions on how to improve this work.

The opinions expressed in this work are those of the author and should not be construed as necessarily representing the opinions of the Rockefeller and Ford foundations, the Lebanon Family Planning Association, or the United Nations. The author is solely responsible for the errors and omissions in this work.

Finally, my deepest gratitude goes to Mary. Both in Lebanon and in the United States, she generously provided me with those very special ingredients that are essential to one's productivity and happiness. To her this book is dedicated.

Beirut, Lebanon Joseph Chamie
January 1981

Introduction: the relevance of religion to fertility

There are a number of reasons why religious affiliation is a particularly worthwhile dimension with which to investigate fertility differentials. First, in many countries (e.g., Ireland, India, Israel, Philippines, Mauritius, and Lebanon) it is a characteristic that has immense social, economic, and political significance. In Lebanon, for example, religious affiliation is the single most important characteristic defining group status. The offices of the president, prime minister, and speaker of the Chamber of Deputies, the composition of the Chamber, and the distribution of government posts are based on religious status.

Second, religious affiliation has considerable theoretical bearing on fertility. A couple's religious status connotes a system of values that can influence fertility via two routes: (1) directly, by imposing sanctions on the practice of birth control or legitimizing the practice of less effective methods only; or (2) indirectly, by indoctrinating its followers with a moral and social philosophy of marriage and family that emphasizes the virtues of reproduction (Westoff 1959, p. 117).

Third, substantial religious differentials in fertility have been empirically documented in a large number of countries. For example, Yaukey (1961) in Lebanon, Rizk (1963) in Egypt, Matras (1973) in Israel, Mazur (1967) in the Soviet Union, Rizk (1973) in Jordan, Sinha (1957) in India, Caldwell (1968) in tropical Africa, and Kirk (1967) in Malaysia, Albania, and Yugoslavia, all found significantly higher fertility rates for Muslims than for non-Muslims.

In the West, religious affiliation has also been found to have a significant effect on fertility. In Europe, Canada, the United States, South Africa, Australia, and New Zealand, studies have shown that Catholics have higher fertility than non-Catholics (Glass 1968; Chou and Brown 1968; Nixon 1963; Burch 1966; Ryder and Westoff 1971; Higgins 1964; Day 1964, 1968). Usually it has been the case that Catholics have higher fertility than Jews or Protestants, with Jews having the lowest fertility of the three groups.

However, there have been puzzling exceptions to this pattern. For instance, Yaukey noted similar fertility levels for Muslims and Christians in rural areas of Lebanon; Rizk (1963) also found this to be the case in rural Egypt. Busia (1954) noted no differences between Muslim and Christian fertility in Ghana. Driver (1963) discovered no significant differences between Muslim and Hindu fertility in India. Also, in an investigation of the 1960 census of Thailand, Goldstein (1970) reported Muslim fertility to be lower than that of either Buddhists or Confucianists.

A possible explanation for such mixed results is that the effect of religion on fertility is generally complicated by the simultaneous effects of other variables that are difficult to adequately control for. In order to properly ascertain the effect of religious affiliation on fertility behavior, a unique body of data is required. As Clark has noted,

> like the other factors, this [religion] also shows considerable inter-correlation with the other variables, and so it is desirable to have cross-tabulations with the other variables controlled. International comparisons clearly do not help here, because so many other variables are involved in them. We can only use data where followers of different religions are living side by side in one country under fairly similar conditions. This consideration alone limits the amount of possible information. (Clark 1967, p. 227)

The 1971 National Fertility and Family Planning survey of Lebanon – a country of considerable religious heterogeneity, with followers of different religions living side by side under reasonably similar conditions – offers a particularly ideal set of data with which to study the effects of religion on fertility. Moreover, confounding effects arising from racial or ethnic differences (such as are found in the United States, Canada, and Australia) are insignificant because the followers of the major faiths in Lebanon differ very little with respect to these characteristics.

1. Theoretical framework

General theoretical model of fertility

The broad determinants of fertility have been delineated by Davis and Blake (1956) and Freedman (1967). These determinants and their relationships to each other and to fertility are illustrated in Figure 1. As fertility as an outcome is the major focus of this investigation, feedback effects that may exist will not be dealt with to any significant extent; attention will be given primarily to those effects that flow from left to right in the figure. Accordingly, fertility is assumed to be directly affected by the levels of the intermediate variables (e.g., age at marriage, use of contraception, and fetal mortality rates); social and economic structure and environmental factors of a population are assumed to affect fertility through their impacts on the intermediate variables. For instance, norms concerning the use of abortion affect fertility indirectly through their influence on the intermediate variables – for example, voluntary fetal mortality – which in turn affect the level of fertility.

Religion is a factor that falls in the domain of the determinant labeled social and economic structure. How religious affiliation is believed to influence fertility is illustrated, in general terms, in Figure 1. According to this model, the effects of religious affiliation operate via the norms about family size and the norms about the intermediate variables, as well as through the intermediate variables themselves. Stated in a slightly different manner, when given appropriate controls for demographic, social, and economic characteristics, fertility differentials between religious groups arise from differences in the intermediate variables, which in turn are due largely to differences in the norms about the intermediate variables and norms about family size.

Explanations for religious differences in fertility

Three major hypotheses have been proposed in the literature to explain religious differences in fertility: (1) the "characteristics" (or "assimila-

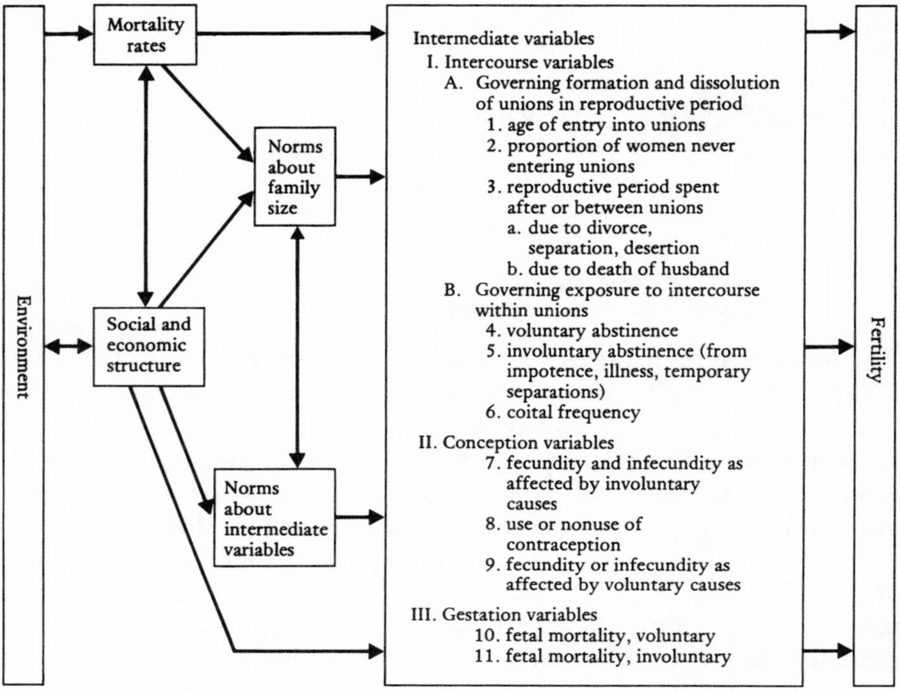

Figure 1. Determinants of fertility.

tionist") hypothesis; (2) the "particularized theology" proposition; and (3) the "minority group status" hypothesis. Advocates of the characteristics hypothesis argue that the religious differentials in fertility are essentially the result of differences in the demographic, social, and economic attributes of the members of the religious groups. Petersen, for example, has aptly summarized the characteristics hypothesis:

> In the process of modernization that the growth of cities and of urban-based social classes effects, one typical consequence is secularization, the tendency of religious-cultural differences to become smaller. Thus, the effect of religion *per se* on the reproductive behavior of most persons in the West is now probably close to nil. What may seem to be a religious influence often reflects the fact that the members of any denomination are typically concentrated in very few places in the social structure as defined by occupation, education, income, or any other of the usual indices. (Petersen 1969, p. 538)

In contrast to the characteristics hypothesis, supporters of the particularized theology proposition contend that the religious differentials in fertility are due to differences in church doctrine. Accordingly, religious groups whose doctrines proscribe the use of contraception and abortion and stress the value of many children should have greater fertility than groups whose doctrines permit contraception and do not emphasize the importance of many children.

The characteristics and particularized theology hypotheses should not be viewed as being mutually exclusive. They are often used to buttress each other:

> If two religious groups do not have explicit or identifiable religious ideologies about birth control or ideal family size, any fertility differences between these religious groups must result from a matrix of social, demographic, and economic characteristics; or in another form, if fertility differences between religious groups persist after controlling for differential social, demographic, and economic characteristics, the explanation of residual fertility differentiation must rest with a particularized religious ideology on birth control and family size. (Goldscheider 1971, p. 273)

Proponents of the third proposition, the minority group status hypothesis, view religious fertility differentials within the larger context of fertility and social organization. They maintain that

> the insecurities of minority group membership operate to depress fertility below majority levels when (1) acculturation of minority groups has occurred in conjunction with the desire for acculturation; (2) equalization of social and economic characteristics occurs and/or social and economic mobility is desired; (3) no pronatalist ideology is associated with the minority group and no norm discourages the use of efficient contraceptives. (Goldscheider 1971, p. 297)

This hypothesis is used to explain not only religious differences in fertility but also ethnic and racial fertility differences (e.g., black–white differences and differences between Japanese-, Chinese-, and Spanish-Americans on the one hand, and Anglo-European–Americans on the other).

Minority group status has generally been defined in terms of the group's size in numbers (e.g., Goldscheider 1971; Kennedy 1973; Sly 1970). Recently, however, Bouvier and Rao (1975) have expanded this definition to include psychological factors. They contend that a group can be a numerical majority and still be a psychological minority, as are the South African blacks. Such groups, they argue, can rid themselves of their minority-status feeling when they perceive (rightly or wrongly) that they have gained entrance into the "Establishment" (p. 186).

Empirically, there is evidence both in support of and against each of these hypotheses. With respect to the characteristics hypothesis, Goldscheider has concluded that fertility differentials between Catholics,

Protestants, and Jews are not merely the consequence of differential social and economic characteristics of these groups.

> Except for some minor qualifications . . . the conclusion of every major empirical study has been that controlling for almost every social and economic characteristic, fertility differences between Protestant, Catholic, and Jewish couples remain. In other words, controlling for race, urban or metropolitan residence, education, occupation, income, and other socioeconomic measures, Catholics retain the lowest levels, and Protestants have an intermediate position. Thus, it cannot be argued that religious differentials in fertility reflect only differential concentrations of these subgroups in socioeconomic or residence categories. The characteristics hypothesis not only fails to admit to the vitality of religious group membership in modern societies but also may be clearly dismissed as inadequate on the basis of empirical evidence now available. (Goldscheider 1971, p. 278)

Empirical support for the characteristics hypothesis comes from a number of studies. For example, in a study of 66 Jewish couples, drawn from the 1955 Growth of American Families Study (Freedman et al. 1959), who were matched with Protestant and Catholic couples along six demographic, socioeconomic dimensions, Freedman, Whelpton, and Smit (1961) found that the controls eliminated the Protestant–Jewish fertility differences, but not the Catholic–Jewish differences. In a very similar study, based on 380 matched Catholic–Protestant couples, Smit (1964) found that the Catholic–Protestant differences in fertility could not be explained by the six factors. These findings seem to suggest that Catholicism had a distinctive effect, but Goldberg (1959) discovered that the religious fertility differentials in Detroit were reduced considerably when analysis was restricted to the purely urban populations: "Catholic–Protestant fertility differences (2.37–2.00) among the two-generation urbanites in Detroit are only at the borderline of statistical significance. The only large religious differentials in fertility for Detroiters are found among the rural migrants" (p. 218).

More recent evidence, however, clearly shows that U.S. Catholic–non-Catholic differentials in fertility and fertility control have become virtually insignificant (Westoff and Ryder 1969; Westoff and Bumpass 1973; Westoff and Jones 1978). For example, in their investigation of the five national fertility surveys of married women, Westoff and Jones concluded that

> the trend toward the convergence which has been in process earlier in the century (Stouffer, 1935) resumed in the mid-sixties and by the approaching mid-seventies . . . has nearly reached unity. In short, the Catholic–non-Catholic differential in

fertility, the distinctiveness of traditionally higher "Catholic" fertility appears to have all but disappeared. (Westoff and Jones 1978, p. 6)

Moreover, Westoff and Jones found that the convergent trends in fertility and fertility control behavior applied to Catholics regardless of their adherence to the norms of the church – that is, to both practicing and nominal Catholics.

The particularized theology hypothesis, which has been commonly used in the explanation of Catholic–non-Catholic fertility differences, is also frequently relied upon to explain Muslim–non-Muslim fertility differentials. For example, in a summary article on Muslim natality, Kirk (1967) argues that Islam has been a more effective barrier to the diffusion of family planning than has Catholicism. The reasons for the high natality of the Muslims, he maintains, are:

1. The high degree of tenacity with which old beliefs and practices are maintained by Muslims
2. The persistent resistance of Muslims to change and to modernity, which are identified with Christianity
3. Conformity to religious and social practices, which are so closely interwoven in Muslim life
4. The strongly patrilinear and patrilocal quality of the Muslim family, with male dominance and responsibility prescribed by the Koran
5. Religious precepts that are favorable to early remarriage of the widowed and divorced
6. The belief that pleasures of flesh, and especially sexual intercourse, are a God-given virtue to be enjoyed and a conjugal obligation to be fulfilled (celibacy is considered abnormal for men and unthinkable for able-bodied women)
7. The unusually subordinate place of women in Muslim society

In contrast, there are others (Sabagh 1970; El-Hamamsy 1972; Saleh 1972; Nazer 1974) who believe differently. For example, El-Hamamsy (1972) feels that greater attention should be given to belief systems on the behavior level and less to Islamic theology; she stresses that there are conditions and factors in Muslim society other than religion that encourage procreation. Omran (1973) also suggests that in order to understand the high fertility of the Muslims, greater emphasis should be placed on the existing conditions in their countries rather than on the doctrines of Islam.

Evidence from studies concerned with minority group status and fertility has been mixed. There are studies that indicate that the fertility of a minority group differs significantly from the fertility of the dominant majority. For example, after analyzing the fertility of Catholics and Protestants on both sides of the Dutch-Belgian and Dutch-German frontiers, Van Heek (1956) concluded that one of the important factors making for high fertility in both areas was the religious élan of the Catholics, which derived from their position as a strong minority. Day (1968) also stressed the minority group status hypothesis in his explanation of Catholic–Protestant differences in New Zealand and Australia. Goldscheider and Uhlenberg (1969) concluded that in the United States, the lower fertility of Jews relative to Protestants and Catholics was not solely the result of differences in the social or economic characteristics of the couples, but was also due to the Jews' minority status. In Northern Ireland and the Republic of Ireland, Kennedy (1973) found minority group status to have an independent effect on fertility when the minority is relatively large, the minority's size is politically important, the minority is economically disadvantaged, and the cohesiveness of the minority is strong. However, he added that "the impact of minority group status on fertility is a less important determinant of fertility than such factors as religion, rural/urban residence, or the selective impact of migration" (p. 85).

There are also studies that have shown the absence of significant differences or a convergence in the fertilities of the majority and minority groups. For example, Van Praag and Lohle-Tart (1974) reported that the previous fertility differentials between Catholics and Protestants in the Netherlands were insignificant by the late sixties. They found that "the 1960's brought a much faster fertility decline in Catholic provinces so that a 16 percent differential in marital fertility around 1960 was more than wiped out by 1967" (p. 304). The aforementioned recent works of Westoff, Ryder, and Bumpass have shown considerable convergence in the fertility of Catholics and Protestants in the United States. Driver (1963) in India, Busia (1954) in Ghana, Yaukey (1961) in rural Lebanon, and Rizk (1963) in rural Egypt all found no significant fertility differences between Muslims and non-Muslims. Taeuber (1955) reported that based on the 1946 census of Cyprus, there was little evidence of substantial differential fertility among the Greek Orthodox and Turkish Muslims (the minority), except possibly at younger ages. Long (1970) noted that Protestant–Jewish fertility differences were nearly insignificant in the big cities of Canada.

He also pointed out that the tendency toward reduction of religious differentials in fertility had been greatest in large cities, uniformly weaker in smaller cities and towns, and weakest in rural areas. A particularly good example of the speed with which a minority group's fertility may converge to the fertility of the majority group is given in the study by Mayer and Marx (1957) of Polish Catholics in Hamtramck, Michigan. They observed that although in 1920 the birthrate of the predominantly immigrant, Polish Catholic community was much above that of the general U.S. population, by 1950 the two rates were very similar.

One general conclusion that seems indicated by the above discussion is that religious fertility differentials are not constant over time. Counries with strong differentials at one time appear to have converging differentials at other times. The framework of explanation for religious differentials in fertility needs to accommodate such trends.

The interaction hypothesis

Based on the preceding review of the literature, it is apparent that none of the three popular hypotheses is entirely adequate in explaining the observed differentials in fertility. In this section a new hypothesis is proposed that is believed to be more generally consistent with the observed differentials and that also provides a broader conceptual framework in which to understand religious differentials in fertility.

This proposition, which I have called the "interaction" hypothesis, maintains that religious differentials in fertility are largely a function of two broad factors: (1) the official doctrines and the current "local orientations" of the religions involved; and (2) the socioeconomic levels of the religious groups. In brief, the theory maintains that there is no single constant effect on fertility that may be attributed to membership in a particular religious group. Religious fertility differentials will depend on the interaction of the socioeconomic levels of the religious groups and the local orientations (by which we mean the current moral attitudes of the religious community) of these groups toward procreation and fertility control. The essence of the hypothesis is shown in Figure 2.

For simplicity, only two religions are shown. The doctrines of Religon I are explicitly pronatalist; they stress the value of many children and consider procreation a religious obligation. Furthermore, they ban the use of birth control techniques. In contrast, the doctrines of Religion II are considerably less pronatalist, and are also not very explicit.

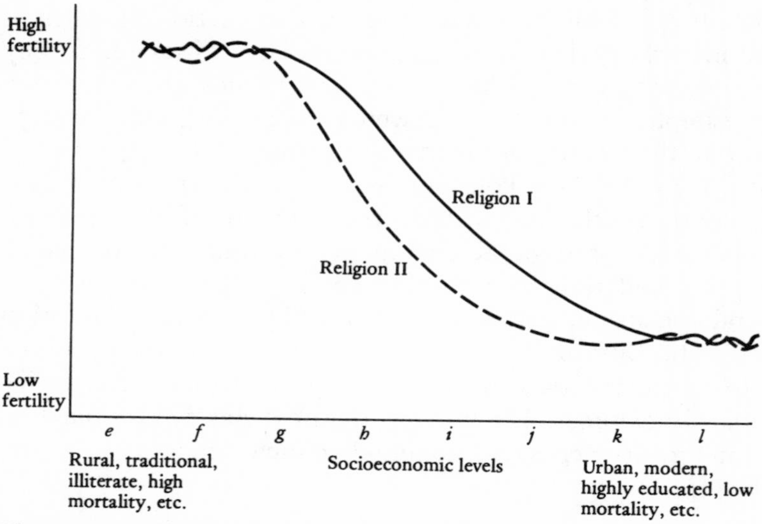

Figure 2. Relationship of religion and fertility.

The use of birth control is permitted and is at the discretion of the couple. At points *e* and *f* on the chart, when both groups are traditional, rural, illiterate, and so forth, the fertility level of both groups is assumed high. Quite apart from any religious doctrines, the social and economic characteristics of this way of life – for example, high mortality, labor intensive agricultural work, and extended family structures – give rise to large family size norms, low average ages at marriage, high proportions of women marrying and remaining in the state of marriage, and little use of contraception and abortion, which in turn promote high levels of fertility for both religious groups.

In fact, under such conditions the doctrines of virtually all the world's major religions are in harmony with high fertility. As Jones and Nortman have concluded,

> since man's struggle for life has been waged against heavy natural odds, it is understandable that Roman Catholicism is not the only major religion to have encouraged a "generous fecundity." The Old Testament stresses fruitfulness in the well known "increase and multiply" verses of Genesis (1:28, 8:17, 9:17). Christianity continued the Old Testament heritage of strong fertility and the Reformation did not modify this tradition. . . the impact of traditional pro-fertility is clearly evident in the major regions of Buddhist, Hindu, and Islamic culture. (Jones and Nortman 1968, p. 2)

Analogously, at points *k* and *l*, when the two groups are modern, educated, urban, and so forth, the fertility of both religious groups is low. Conformity to pronatalist religious doctrines is suppressed or overcome by the characteristics of modern society. Religion is simply no longer an important determinant of fertility behavior in such a modern society; other variables or characteristics such as education, residence status, and occupation are the overriding variables. These characteristics bring about changes such as small family size ideals, greater spacing between births, high average ages at marriage, and widespread use of and reliance on contraceptives and/or abortion, which in turn lead to lower levels of fertility for the two religious groups. Regardless of religious affiliation, groups that are urban, experience low mortality, maintain equality between the sexes, and so forth, will have low fertility. However, a period of time may be necessary before the religious differences converge, because strong religious and cultural values that influence life-styles may have some persistent effect for a time even under modernized conditions.

In contrast, fertility differentials will be observed for those clusters of couples existing at levels between those mentioned above. From points *f* to *k*, the adherents of Religion I maintain consistently higher levels of fertility than those believing in Religion II. Why should this be the case? The fundamental reason is that members of the more pronatalist groups do not adjust as quickly to the new pressures and realities of the changing society. Pronatalist customs and attitudes are reinforced by the doctrines of Religion I so that change is less rapid. Due to the greater stress and concern placed on such matters by their religion's orientation, these couples cling relatively more tenaciously to the fertility-related values and behavior of lower socioeconomic levels, such as large family size ideals, low average age at marriage, little spacing between births, and low usage of contraception. As a consequence, members of Religion I do not and/or cannot maintain levels of fertility similar to followers of Religion II.

In brief, the interaction hypothesis maintains that religious values and orientations that are pronatalist have their principal effect during the demographic transition because their influence produces a lag in the adjustment of their adherents' fertility to the new conditions for which low fertility is an appropriate response. Before the demographic transition high fertility is appropriate for everyone, so religious affiliation does not differentiate. After the transition, the religious influence is eventually negated by the conditions of modern society.

2. Data and methodology

Data

Research dealing with the Lebanese population is usually of two sorts. Purely descriptive studies constitute the bulk of the material. These studies report percentages, frequencies, rates, and so forth, and are usually based on small nonprobability samples chosen from a school, hospital, village, or city. Only the more significant descriptive studies based on reasonably good samples are discussed here; others are listed in the References. A different type of research is oriented toward the investigation and explanation of demographic phenomena. Until recently, the study by Yaukey (1961) was the only one that dealt with the explanation of Lebanese fertility behavior. Consequently, the results of Yaukey's study will be examined closely.

One of the earliest nongovernmental inquiries was conducted by Churchill (1954). His main objective was to obtain a socioeconomic profile of Beirut. From his stratified, random sample of 1,903 households in Beirut, he was able to put together a general description of the household structure that existed at the time. One of his important findings was that plural marriages were rare; of the 1,903 marriages, only two were plural. A second noteworthy finding concerned the unusually high proportion of male children in the households:

> It would appear that there is a significant difference in the incidence of children remaining in the household by sex. It is possible that there is a survival differential in favor of male children, but on the other hand, there is also a greater tendency for male children to remain in the household.[1] (Churchill 1954, p. 5)

In 1965, Churchill and Sabbagh (1968) carried out a study of Beirut that was somewhat similar to Churchill's earlier one. One of the most obvious changes found was the great increase in the use of modern appliances. Electric refrigerators, radios, washing machines, electric irons, and so forth, had become common possessions of families in Beirut. With respect to the family, a strong trend toward egalitarianism was noted. Patterns of interrelationships within the family had become more modern and egalitarian - due, in great part no doubt, to the improvement in the status of women.

> The *patria potestas* has been whittled down steadily between 1952 and 1965, and women in the middle classes are assuming roles of partners as their educational level approaches that of men. The bride price among Moslems and the dowry among Christians are becoming nominal and are continued in many cases as a bow to tradition. More women are working and in more categories of job opportunity. Office personnel is becoming female with the government lagging behind the private sector but yielding slowly. More women are training for the professions except in medicine. (Churchill and Sabbagh 1968, p. 49)

Limited descriptive demographic information may also be gained from a study by Prothro and Diab (1974). For example, on the basis of an inquiry into Sunni (a major Muslim sect) religious court records in the Lebanese cities of Sidon and Tripoli during the period from 1920 to 1965, they tentatively concluded that age at marriage in Lebanon has been increasing for women and remaining about the same for men. Also, from a quota sample of about 300 households in Beirut and Tripoli, they found that Sunnis prefer sons rather than daughters, and that their ideal family size is approximately four children.

Until 1971 virtually all existing information and knowledge concerning fertility and family planning in Lebanon and in the Levant came from the 1957-58 study by Yaukey (1961). Unfortunately, because he could obtain only a relatively small nonprobability sample, and because he used gross categories of important variables, the generalizability and value of Yaukey's work are limited. Because of political difficulties in Lebanon at the time, Yaukey was unable to secure a good sample. His sample consisted of 909 couples purposively drawn from four of the 40 districts of Beirut, and from two rural villages, one predominately Muslim and the other Christian. Yaukey's study was not descriptive, but explanatory in intent: "The goal was not to describe the fertility of Lebanon as a whole, but rather to point out interrelationships between fertility and other characteristics for a cross-section of Lebanese women" (p. 16). Yaukey did not measure fertility in particular time intervals - for example, in annual birthrates - but rather focused on the total fertility of particular women.

Yaukey's analysis could not adequately deal with some of the main issues that he addressed. For example, the measures of socioeconomic status that he attempted to relate to fertility behavior were very gross:

(1) education - both husband and wife illiterate versus either illiterate; (2) rooms per capita - 0.6 or less versus 0.7 or more; (3) husband's occupation - farmer versus nonfarmer. Consequently, his conclusions involving socioeconomic status must be viewed as tentative.

The main conclusions of his analyses may be summarized as follows:

1. No significant religious fertility differences existed for the sects of Islam (i.e., between Sunnis, Shi'as, and Druzes), or for the denominations of Christianity (i.e., between the Maronites, other Catholics, and Orthodox Christians).
2. Urban fertility depended on religion, whereas rural fertility did not. Urban Christians demonstrated considerably lower fertility than did urban Muslims, although, in contrast, rural Christians demonstrated essentially the same fertility as did rural Muslims.
3. City dwellers showed lower fertility than did those living in the rural areas. The fertility rates of both religious groups in the villages were quite high.
4. For Muslims, residence did not significantly affect fertility, but for Christians, city residence lowered fertility (i.e., urban Christians had 69 percent lower fertility than rural Christians).
5. The influences of urban residence and high socioeconomic status on fertility appeared to operate independently.
6. A secondary fertility differential was a socioeconomic one among the urban Muslims; however, it was not as important for urban Christians.
7. In the village, no fertility differences by socioeconomic status were found in either religious group.
8. With few exceptions, the same fertility patterns seemed to have applied both to women in the older generation and women in the younger generation.

Throughout this study, Yaukey's findings will be closely compared to my results.

A 1970 survey (WHO 1976) conducted by investigators at the School of Public Health of the American University of Beirut also contains some information on Lebanese religious fertility differentials. The study was a comparison of two religious groups, Shi'a Muslim and Maronite Christian, living in the Beirut suburbs of Mreiyje, Chiah, and Ghebeiri. It was based on a stratified, cluster sample of neighborhoods in the three suburbs and consisted of 3,004 married women (1,545 Shi'a and 1,459 Maronite) under 45 years of age with husband living at home.

As did Yaukey's work, this study suffered from two major weaknesses: nonprobability sampling techniques and inadequate controls for socioeconomic characteristics. Because the study is based on quota sampling techniques, one cannot properly generalize to the larger Shi'a and Maronite communities, as the results may simply represent differences between the neighborhoods chosen rather than true differences between the larger religious groups.

The lack of sufficient controls for the substantial background differences between the two religious groups opens to serious question a number of the conclusions that the authors present. For instance, although the groups were divided into middle and low social status categories, this was not at all adequate for comparative purposes. Specifically, for example, whereas the proportions illiterate among middle- and low-status Shi'a women were 65 and 94 percent, respectively, they were 43 and 83 percent, respectively, for middle- and low-status Maronite women. Also, although the proportions whose husbands were unskilled workers were 12 and 53 percent among middle- and low-status Shi'a women, the proportions were 4 and 27 percent for middle- and low-status Maronite women.

Nevertheless, for the sake of completeness as well as for comparative purposes, we briefly summarize the major relevant findings of the study.

1. On the average, Shi'a women married earlier than Maronite women.
2. Among Shi'as and Maronites, the higher the level of education, the later the marriage age.
3. Although fertility varied little by social class within each sect, the fertility of the Shi'as was greater than that of the Maronites (e.g., the number of children ever born for age group 40–44 was 9.7 for Shi'as and 6.5 for Maronites).
4. The average number of children considered ideal by all women was about six, with little variation by religion, social class, wife's occupation, or parity of the woman's mother.
5. Mortality for children under five years of age was higher for Shi'as than for Maronites. In addition, among Shi'as, child mortality rates were higher in the low-status than in the middle-status group.
6. Nearly 85 percent of the Shi'as and Maronites approved of birth control.

7. More Shiʻa than Maronite women disapproved of birth control for religious reasons (which is contrary to expectations, as Islam does not oppose birth control, although the Roman Catholic Church does).
8. Higher proportions of Maronite than of Shiʻa women either had used or were using birth control.
9. For Shiʻas there was an increase in birth control use with educational level (58 percent with no schooling, 69 percent with primary schooling, and 73 percent with secondary or higher practiced birth control), but for Maronites the trend was slightly in the opposite direction (85, 80, and 79 percent, respectively).
10. At the time of the survey, the four most commonly used birth control methods and their percentages for each religious group were (1) Shiʻas: coitus interruptus, 18 percent; oral pill, 11 percent; condom, 6 percent; rhythm, 4 percent; and (2) Maronites: coitus interruptus, 42 percent; oral pill, 8 percent; condom, 9 percent; rhythm, 10 percent.

Since Lebanon's independence from the French in 1943, there have been three major government-sponsored demographic inquiries into the composition of the Lebanese population. The first, done by Gibb (1948), was based mainly on the 1943 "Mira Census," which was designed primarily for rationing purposes. The Mira Census was not truly a census of the Lebanese population; the last genuine census of the population was done in 1932 during the French Mandate. Gibb's findings were extremely general and did not yield any specific demographic estimates. Gibb's appraisal of Lebanon's vital statistics was particularly noteworthy: "It is not considered that available statistics of births and deaths are sufficiently accurate to be used. In fact, it is felt that they give an erroneous picture" (p. 3). Although made over twenty-five years ago, his statement is still applicable today.

During the early sixties, there was another attempt to make the demographic estimates needed for developmental plans; this work was conducted under the auspices of the Ministry of Planning (République Libanaise 1960). Not surprisingly, given the delicate situation concerning the religiopolitical composition of Lebanon, only the most general demographic information resulted from this work – for example, population size, geographic distribution, and economic conditions.

In contrast to these two earlier works, data from the stratified, cluster sample consisting of about 30,000 households carried out in

1970 (*L'enquête par Sondage sur la Population Active au Liban*, République Libanaise 1972, hereafter referred to as the *PAL* survey) provided a variety of basic demographic information – for example, age-sex structure, marital status, and geographic, educational, and economic distributions by sex and age. For the first time in the history of modern-day Lebanon, a variety of reasonably accurate demographic estimates (e.g., proportion employed, proportion illiterate, number employed by age and sex, population distribution by place of birth and current residence, and marital status by age and sex) is available for the Lebanese population. One striking, but no doubt intended, shortcoming of the *PAL* study, however, is that it did not ask about religious affiliation.

More specifically, the *PAL* survey was based on a stratified, two-stage cluster sample of dwellings. The sampling frame was an updated version of the official list of villages and towns drawn up in 1964. Places were stratified by size: (1) Beirut and surroundings; (2) other main towns; (3) places with populations of 1,000 to 9,999; and (4) places with less than 1,000 inhabitants. All places with populations of 10,000 or more were selected, and 142 villages were chosen at random strata three and four. The sampling fractions of the first stage were 100 percent for strata one and two, 32.20 percent for stratum three, and 6.67 percent in stratum four. The second stage consisted of selecting the dwellings. The sampling fractions in the second stage were chosen so that an overall sampling of one-fifteenth was obtained for each stratum. A systematic sampling procedure was used to select the dwellings in the localities.

Using the households from the *PAL* survey as a sampling frame, the Lebanon Family Planning Association (LFPA) selected a 10 percent subsample for an inquiry into fertility and family planning patterns in Lebanon. This subsample (hereafter referred to as the *NFFP* survey) was the first national fertility and family planning survey of the Lebanese population. The *NFFP* survey, involving interviews with 2,795 currently married women between 15 and 49 years old, provides the basic data for this investigation.

The interviewing, conducted in Arabic with husbands not present, was done in the summer of 1971 by social workers who were under the supervision of the LFPA. All the social workers were given a training course in interviewing before they began their assignments. The coding, punching, and editing were done under the author's supervision at a private computer agency in Beirut.

The interaction hypothesis and the NFFP data

Because the data under investigation are taken from a society at a single point in time, we should not expect to encounter the entire pattern of religious fertility differentials (that is, from no differences, to differences, to no differences). On the contrary, examining data of this kind permits the observation of only a portion of the total pattern.[2] The portion observed depends to a large extent on the stage of development of the country and the degree of socioeconomic diversity among its population. For instance, if the data were to refer to an area at a high economic level (e.g., Western Europe, the United States, Japan), then one might observe only differentials similar to those on the right-hand side of the pattern shown in Figure 1 (points *j, k, l*). In contrast, if the data were to come from a society at a relatively low level of development with most of its population living at a low socioeconomic level (e.g., Bangladesh), then differentials similar to those on the left-hand side of the pattern might generally be observed (points *e, f, g*). Or, if the data were from a society at an intermediate stage of development with a relatively high degree of socioeconomic diversity among its population (possibly, for example, Iran or Brazil), then religious fertility differentials like those in the middle section of the pattern might be encountered (points *i* to *k*).

As Lebanon is a society at an intermediate stage of development with a relatively high degree of socioeconomic diversity among its population, we should expect to observe religious differentials in fertility like those in the middle section of the pattern of Figure 2. Differentials like those for point *i* to *e* ought not to be encountered among the Lebanese due to the near absence of particularly low socioeconomic levels such as are generally found in rural areas of Bangladesh and India. According to the interaction hypothesis, after controlling for demographic differences such as marriage duration, wife's age, and residence status, religious differentials in fertility for the Lebanese should be greatest among the lower socioeconomic classes and smallest among the higher socioeconomic classes, with religious groups with the more pronatalist orientations having the higher fertility. In other words, one should not expect to find socioeconomic status operating similarly on the fertilities of the different religious groups; rather, one should expect to find a significant interaction effect. The relationship of socioeconomic status to fertility is expected to differ as a function of the orientations of the religious groups. If, however, the interaction is minor (that is, if the interaction hypothesis is incorrect), then a model stipulating a constant effect of religious affiliation operating across all socioeconomic categories ought to be employed to determine the specific effects of religious status on fertility as well as its effect in relationship to the other explanatory variables. In other words, if the interaction hypothesis is not consistent with the *NFFP* results, then the results will be considered vis-à-vis the characteristics, particularized theology, and minority group status hypotheses.

Similar strategies of analysis will be utilized to investigate the probable sources of the religious fertility differentials, namely, differences in the number of children wanted and differences in the willingness and ability to control fertility. Again, the objectives are to determine whether or not there is a significant interaction effect, and then to develop a model that takes account of this interaction, if it exists, and that specifies the impact of religious affiliation on the dependent variables in relationship to the other independent variables.

Statistical techniques

Most of the major analyses in this research involve a problem having the form of a quantitative dependent variable and two or more independent variables (which may be quantitative or qualitative), with the objective being to establish the relationships between the independent variables and the dependent variable. Among the repertoire of statistical techniques available to the social scientist, multiple classification analysis (MCA) is a method that is not only suited for this type of problem, but also seems particularly appropriate given the issues being considered in this investigation.

MCA is a technique for determining the interrelationships between a number of explanatory variables and a dependent variable within the context of an additive model (Andrews et al. 1973). It assesses simultaneously how several explanatory variables determine a dependent variable. The method permits the researcher to obtain: (1) the net effects of an independent variable on the dependent variable; that is, the deviations of the category mean from the grand mean after adjusting for the effects of other predictors; and (2) the proportion of the variance in the dependent variable explained by one or more of the predictors.

The statistical model is as follows:

$$Y_{ijk\ldots} = \bar{Y} + a_i + b_j + \ldots + e_{ijk\ldots}$$

where

$Y_{ijk\ldots}$ = the value on the dependent variable for individual k who belongs to category i of predictor A, category j of predictor B, etc.

$\bar{Y}$ = the grand mean of the dependent variable

a_i = the effect of belonging to the ith category of predictor A.

b_j = the effect of belonging to the jth category of predictor B.

$e_{ijk\ldots}$ = the error term for individual k.

The model maintains that the score of each person (or each unit of analysis) on the dependent variable may be treated as a sum of coefficients assigned to each of the categories characterizing the individual (or the unit of analysis), plus the grand mean, plus an error term.

If the predictors are orthogonal, that is, noncorrelated, then the coefficients are simply the observed deviations of the category means from the grand mean. With nonorthogonal predictors, that is, correlated predictors, the coefficients represent the deviations of the category means from the grand mean after adjusting for the effects of the other predictors in the equation. The adjusted coefficients are arrived at by minimizing the sum of squared errors, and also by assuming that the sum of the coefficients (weighted for the number of cases) should equal zero for each predictor.

Essentially, MCA is a multiple regression technique using dummy variables with the only difference being in the form of the output. Whereas in MCA the coefficients are expressed as deviations from the grand mean, the coefficients in dummy variable regression are usually expressed as deviations from a constant term based on a composite sum of the means of the excluded subclasses.

A major strength of MCA is that is makes no assumptions of linearity or monotonicity as to the form of the relationship of the dependent variable to any of the explanatory variables. Thus, the order of the categories for a predictor is generally not utilized when obtaining the solution, although it may be useful for interpreting the results.

The dependent variable may be intervally or dichotomously scaled. If intervally scaled, it should not be seriously skewed, for being so unduly affects the values of the means and variances. Most of our intervally scaled dependent variables are reasonably symmetrical, and therefore this condition does not pose a serious problem.

When the dependent variable is dichotomously scaled, there are a number of possible technical difficulties (Goodman 1973; Nerlove and Press 1973). For example, the disturbance terms are likely to be heteroscedastic, and therefore least squares estimates will lead to inefficient estimators and imprecise predictors. Also, values may be produced that are greater than one or less than zero. Because the interval goes from zero to one, this is obviously unacceptable.

However, when the dichotomous variable is not severely skewed – that is, when it is between 0.2 and 0.8 – these difficulties are minimal. In addition, alternate methods would also have their own problems. For instance, the use of log-linear model techniques would be problematic given the extremely large number of zero cells that would be generated using our independent variables. Consequently, we utilize ordinary least squares regression techniques with dichotomous dependent variables, but indicate when the results of the analyses are tenuous or likely to be misleading.

The principal weakness of the MCA technique is that it is insensitive to the presence of interaction. The additive model assumes that there is an effect for belonging to category *i* of predictor *A*, category *j* of predictor *B*, and so forth but no additional effect for belonging to any particular combination of the categories. If the case exists where the effect of one predictor on the dependent variable depends to a significant extent on the level of another predictor, we will be unable to detect this using MCA, and therefore will be incorrectly specifying the relationships between the explanatory variables and the dependent variable. However, because we are anticipating certain interaction effects (e.g., the effect of education on fertility will depend on religious affiliation), it will be possible to test for their presence and significance.

Our test for interaction will be based on dummy variable multiple regression primarily because it permits the specification of main effects and interaction terms. Again, both interval and nominal scale variables may be utilized in the model. In contrast to MCA, the interval scale variables remain intervally scaled. However, nominal scale variables are treated as they were in MCA. They are arbitrarily converted to variables having the simple scores of 0 and 1 – that is, to dummy variables. For example, for our five religious groups we would have the following four dummy variables:

$$
\begin{aligned}
Z_1 &= 1 \text{ if respondent is Catholic} \\
&= 0 \text{ otherwise} \\
Z_2 &= 1 \text{ if respondent is non-Catholic Christian} \\
&= 0 \text{ otherwise} \\
Z_3 &= 1 \text{ if respondent is Sunni} \\
&= 0 \text{ otherwise} \\
Z_4 &= 1 \text{ if respondent is Druze} \\
&= 0 \text{ otherwise}
\end{aligned}
$$

There is no need for Z_5 for Shi'a because when Z_1, Z_2, Z_3, and Z_4 are all known, we know the value of Z_5. For instance, when they are all 0, then the respondent is Shi'a.

Dummy variable multiple regression produces a variety of coefficients – for example, coefficients for main effects, interaction effects, multiple correlation coefficients, and so forth. Although we will be interested in the values of these coefficients, our primary concern will be with testing for the significance of the increase in the explained sum of squares due to the addition of the interaction terms. On the one hand, if we find that the increase is not significant, then we are justified in concluding that the interaction terms are minor and may be left out of the model. On the other hand, if the interaction terms lead to a significant increase in the explained sum of squares, then these variables should be included in the model.

The test for the significance of interaction will be an F test, that is, a comparison of the interaction sum of squares with the error sum of squares, adjusted for their respective degrees of freedom:

$$F = \frac{(R_i^2 - R_a^2)/(k_i - k_a)}{(1 - R_i^2)/(N - k_i - 1)}$$

where

R^2 = percentage of the variance explained
N = the total number of cases
k = the number of independent variables in the model
i = the interaction model
a = the additive model

The assumptions for the application of dummy variable regression are independent random sampling, and normally distributed disturbance term with constant variance. It is unlikely that the Lebanese data fully meet all these requirements. Therefore, during the analyses in the following chapters, an attempt will be made to inform the reader of serious departures from these assumptions and to indicate how these violations may be expected to affect the results and interpretations.

3. Lebanese religious groups

Although there are approximately seventeen religious sects in Lebanon, the *NFFP* survey distinguishes between five major religious groups: among the Muslims, (1) Sunnis, (2) Shi'as (also known as Mutawalis in Lebanon), and (3) Druzes;[1] and among the Christians, (4) Catholics, and (5) non-Catholic Christians. The Catholic group consists of members of the following sects: Maronite, Greek Catholic, Armenian Catholic, Syrian Catholic, Latin, and Chaldean. The non-Catholic Christian group is made up of four sects: Greek Orthodox, Armenian Orthodox, Protestant, and Syrian Orthodox. Minor sects and couples stating no religious preference are categorized separately. However, because they constituted less than 1 percent of the sample, they are excluded from most of the analyses.

As may be observed in Table 1, the Catholic and non-Catholic Christian groups consist predominately of one or two sects.[2] Roughly 80 percent of the Catholic group are Maronites.[3] The second largest sect among the Catholics is the Greek Catholic, which constitutes about 15 percent of the Catholic group. The non-Catholic Christian group consists mainly of members of the Greek Orthodox and Armenian Orthodox sects. They represent approximately 65 and 29 percent, respectively, of the entire non-Catholic Christian group.

Before discussing the positions of the five religious groups on procreation and fertility control, I shall briefly mention noteworthy doctrinal distinctions among the sects of the two major faiths and present a short discussion of Lebanon's recent history and relevant aspects of its social, economic, and political structures.[4] My aims in doing so are to provide a brief explanation for those readers who are not generally familiar with Lebanon, to highlight some of the important linkages that exist between the demography of the population and the sociopolitical system, and to describe significant socioeconomic differentials that exist among the religious groups.

Table 1. *Enumerated population of Lebanon in 1922 and 1932 and estimates for 1943, 1951, and 1956 by religion*

Religion	Year 1922	1932	1943	1951	1956
Muslim	273,366	383,180	495,003	571,109	624,434
Sunni	124,786	175,925	222,594	271,734	285,698
Shi'a	104,947	154,208	200,698	237,107	250,605
Druze	43,633	53,047	71,711	62,268	88,131
Alawi	—[a]	—	—	—	—
Isma'li	—	—	—	—	—
Christian	355,668	392,544	544,822	700,154	769,558
Catholic					
Maronite	199,182	226,378	318,201	377,544	423,708
Greek Catholic	42,426	45,999	61,956	81,764	87,788
Armenian Catholic		5,964	—	14,218	14,622
Syrian Catholic	12,651[b]	2,675	—	5,911	5,699
Latin (Roman)		—	—	4,127	4,506
Chaldean		528	—	1,390	1,466
Non-Catholic					
Greek Orthodox	81,409	76,522	106,658	130,858	148,927
Armenian Orthodox		25,462	58,007	67,139	63,679
Protestant		6,712	—	12,641	14,365
Syrian Orthodox		2,574	—	4,562	4,798
Other					
Jew, Baha'i, etc.	—	9,819	6,596	12,677	13,876
Population	629,034	785,543	1,046,421	1,303,940	1,407,868

[a] The dash indicates that no figure had been given in the original source.
[b] This figure refers to all Christians other than Maronites, Greek Orthodox, and Greek Catholics.
Sources: 1922 and 1932: official census figures, cited in Himadeh. 1936, pp. 408–9, and also discussed in Hourani, 1946. 1943: official estimates, cited in Hourani, 1946, p. 121. 1951: estimates by Tabbarah, 1954. 1956: estimates cited in *An-Nahar* (Beirut), no. 6249, April 26, 1956, and also discussed in Zuwiyya-Yamak, 1966, p. 27.

Doctrinal distinctions

The chief division within Islam is between the Sunnis and the other sects.[5] The Sunnis, who represent roughly 90 percent of the Muslims of the world, regard themselves as followers of the original Islamic orthodoxy, as set forth not only in the Koran, but also in the Hadiths (a collection of narratives based on the customs, sayings, and deeds of the Prophet Mohammed and his Companions) and in the system of theology and jurisprudence built up by the major Islamic thinkers. The Shi'as constitute the second largest major sect of Islam. There are two fundamental, interrelated differences between the Sunnis and the Shi'as; these differences have to do with succession and interpretation. After the death of the Prophet Mohammed in 632 A.D., the question arose of who should become leader. The Sunnis took the position that the leader should be elected; the Shi'as, in contrast, believed that the leader should come from the family of the Prophet. Furthermore, the Shi'as believed that this leader, or Imam, should interpret and explain the divine message according to the requirements and needs of the time.

These issues became a serious problem and led to a schism later in the same century. The Shi'as maintain that the succession to the Prophet passed not to the orthodox line of caliphs whom the Sunnis recognize, but to a hereditary line of Imams who were both the spiritual and the temporal heads of Islam, and of whom the first was Ali. The majority of the Shi'as also recognize twelve Imams, the last of whom disappeared in the ninth century, but is expected to reappear in the future.

The Druze sect developed in the eleventh century as an offshoot of the Isma'li faction of Shi'a Islam in Egypt under the Fatimid Caliph Hakim, whom the Druzes believe is the last Imam. Within the Islamic community, the Druzes differ significantly from the Sunnis and Shi'as (Makarem 1974). Doctrinally, they believe in the ideas of successive incarnations of God and the transmigration of souls. They have their own scriptures, which are based to a large extent on the Koran. Their laws regarding domestic relations are distinct from those of the Sunnis and Shi'as. For example, they forbid polygamy and make divorce considerably more difficult to obtain than do either of the other two Muslim sects. Such differences have led some observers to conclude that the status of women is higher among Druzes than among Sunnis or Shi'as (Baer 1966, p. 82).

The major division within Christianity that we will be concerned with is the Catholic versus non-Catholic Christian distinction. The Catholics are mostly members of the Uniate churches (i.e., Eastern Christian churches in union with the Roman Catholic church, but with their own rites, customs, and so forth. They recognize papal supremacy, but maintain their own liturgies and certain distinctive organizational features. Most of the Catholics in Lebanon (roughly 80 percent) are Maronites. The Maronite church, founded in about 700 A.D., originally held the monothelite doctrine that Jesus had two natures, human and divine, but one divine will. In the twelfth century they relinquished this doctrine, and in the fifteenth century they united with Rome.

The non-Catholic Christians are predominately members of the Eastern Orthodox church, which separated from the Western church in the eleventh century. Of the several doctrinal differences between the two churches, one of the most important is the one dealing with the Procession of the Holy Ghost. Eastern Orthodoxy maintains that the Holy Spirit proceeds only "from the Father"; the Roman Catholic church believes that the Holy Spirit proceeds "from the Son" as well as from the Father (Rosten 1975, p. 115). Another important difference, which is of greater concern to us, is that the Eastern church does not accept the supremacy of the Pope; it considers only the church as a whole to be infallible. The Greek Orthodox, who make up about two-thirds of the non-Catholic Christians in Lebanon, are subject to the jurisdiction of the Patriarch of Antioch, and their liturgical language is Arabic.

The Armenian Orthodox (Gregorians) are the second largest non-Catholic Christian sect; they constitute roughly 29 percent of the non-Catholics. They believe in the Monophysite doctrine that Christ has only a divine nature, and not also a human nature. The Gregorian church has an Armenian liturgy. It has five patriarchs, of which the Catholicos of Echmiadzin is the most honored.

Social, economic, and political characteristics

Throughout Lebanon's modern history, religious affiliation and the distribution of the members of the various religious sects have played increasingly important roles.[6] Smock and Smock note that during the seventeenth, eighteenth, and nineteenth centuries

> social and economic differentiations played important roles in Lebanese history, but it was confessional identification that was the most clearly, most consistently, and most self-consciously defined. The most serious confessional conflict in Lebanon took place from 1840–1860, culminating in the Druze-Christian civil war of 1860. Even in periods of less overt conflict, confessional identity usually constituted the principal axis of collective activity, and this was especially the case from about 1800 onwards. (Smock and Smock 1975, p. 30)

Khalaf (1978a) also points out that in the nineteenth century, in order to avoid political subordination of one sect by another, successive efforts were made with regard to the geographic reorganization of the area's administrative divisions as well as to the numerical rearrangement of the population for the basis of representation. More specifically, Khalaf writes:

> The partition scheme of 1843 divided Mount Lebanon into administrative districts: a northern district administered by a Maronite governor (qa'immaqam), and a southern district administered by a Druze; the Reglement of Shakib Efendi of 1845; and the Reglement Organique of 1861 following the civil war of 1860 were all, among other things, efforts to institutionalize confessional representation . . . As confessional representation became rooted into the political system, demographic variables assumed more prominence. (Khalaf 1978a, pp. 1–2)

It should be mentioned that the sense of separateness and distrust among the religious communities was not simply a matter of Muslim versus Christian; differentiation among the Christians (primarily among Maronites, Greek Orthodox, Greek Catholics, and Roman Catholics) and among Muslims (primarily among Sunnis, Shi'as, and Druzes) was nearly as great as that between the two major faiths (Smock and Smock 1975, p. 29).

At the beginning of the twentieth century, the territory of Lebanon was still under the control of the Ottomans. At that time, "Lebanon" referred to Mount Lebanon, an area restricted approximately to the Lebanon mountain range and extending as far north and south as Tripoli and Sidon, respectively, but not including these two cities.[7]

The population of Mount Lebanon in 1900 was about 400,000; the majority were Maronites (Table 2). According to the 1895 estimates of Cuinet (1896) and the 1913 Ottoman census of Mount Lebanon, about 57 percent of the population was Maronite; 12–14 percent was Greek Orthodox; 11–12 percent was Druze; and 7–9 percent was Greek Catholic. Taken as a whole, Christians constituted about 80 percent of the population, with the Sunnis and Shi'as representing no more than half of the Muslim population.

After the defeat of the Ottomans, the Allied Supreme Council gave mandatory control of Mount Lebanon and Greater Syria to France. Seeking to strengthen the political position and economic viability of Mount Lebanon's pro-French Maronite Christian community, the French annexed to Mount Lebanon (at Syria's expense) the coastal regions of Tripoli, Beirut, Sidon, and Tyre, and the Bekaa plain, areas

Table 2. *Estimated population of Mount Lebanon in 1895 and enumerated population in 1913 by religion*

Religion	1895	1913
Muslim	80,234	85,232
Sunni	13,576	14,529
Shi'a	16,846	23,413
Druze	49,812	47,290
Christian	319,296	329,482
Maronite	229,680	242,308
Greek Catholic	34,472	31,936
Greek Orthodox	54,208	52,356
Other Christian	936	2,882
Population	399,530	414,747

Sources: 1895 figures: Cuinet (1896), discussed in Courbage and Fargues (1974); 1913 figures: Courbage and Fargues (1974).

that were populated mainly by Muslims. And on September 1, 1920, the French representative, General Henri Gouraud, officially declared the establishment of the State of Greater Lebanon.

This new country, which is essentially modern Lebanon, was roughly 100 percent larger in land area and 50 percent more populated than Mount Lebanon. Greater Lebanon's religious composition also differed substantially from Mount Lebanon's. Whereas Mount Lebanon consisted overwhelmingly of Maronite Christians, Greater Lebanon's population reportedly had only a slight Christian majority (Table 1). With the Christians being in the majority as well as being decidedly favored by the governing French authorities, the Muslims in the newly annexed territories became increasingly resentful of the French and Lebanese Christians.

The structure of the Lebanese republic was influenced greatly by precedents set up under the Ottoman rule as well as by the French governmental system. According to the Lebanese constitution, the Chamber of Deputies is elected by the population in such a manner that it is proportionately representative of the various confessional communities. Throughout Lebanon's history this proportion has remained unchanged in the ratio of six Christians to five Muslims; consequently, the total number of deputies must be divisible by eleven – for example, forty-four deputies in 1952, sixty-six in 1957, and ninety-nine in 1960 to the present. The president is in turn elected by a two-thirds majority of the deputies for a term of six years and is eligible for reelection only after a span of six additional years. The president then chooses a prime minister who is responsible for forming a cabinet. To remain in power, the cabinet needs a vote of confidence from the Chamber of Deputies; a vote of no confidence, however, is a constitutional right that is rarely exercised. A cabinet generally falls as a result of internal dissension or because the president withdraws his backing.

It should be emphasized that although the Chamber is intended to be representative of the confessional communities, there are no similar constitutional provisions requiring that the offices of the president, prime minister, and cabinet members be assigned on the basis of religious status. However, these offices are assigned by religious status according to the National Pact of 1943, which was a verbal accord reached by the Maronite leader Bisharah al-Khouri and the Sunni leader Riyad al-Sulh.[8] This agreement spelled out the basic roles of the religious groups in the government as well as the relationships Lebanon would maintain with Western Arab nations. A crucial ingredient of the pact was the provision that in the future, as had been the tradition in the past, presidents would be Maronites (the largest single sect according to the 1932 census), prime ministers would be Sunnis (the second largest sect), speakers of the Chamber of Deputies would be Shiʿas (the third largest sect), and so forth.[9]

Despite the Lebanese constitution's stipulation that the government would be proportionately representative of the sizes of the various religious sects, it lacks an explicit definition of the procedure by which the representative proportions are to be determined. Are the proportions to be based only on those Lebanese who reside in Lebanon? Or only on those Lebanese who have their permanent residence in Lebanon? Or on all Lebanese citizens and their children regardless of place of residence? As it is estimated that there are somewhere near 5 million "Lebanese" living outside Lebanon, as compared to about 2.5 million living in Lebanon, an acceptable definition of the Lebanese population is much more than an academic question. This ambiguity has been a continuous source of friction among the various Lebanese religiopolitical groups and is the primary reason why the Lebanese have attempted to avoid many political and constitutional issues by not conducting a census.

In brief, the Lebanese political system is an unusual mixture of traditional and secular features. At first glance and from a distance, the country has the image of a state based on democratic institutions and liberal doctrines; yet, upon closer inspection, one finds that the country is far from this kind of state. The country's parties, parliamentary coalitions, blocs, and various pressure groups run along religious, communal, and personal lines to such an extent that the interests of the larger society are often put in a secondary position, if not thwarted altogether.

These political features of Lebanon are reinforced by the existence of sharp and deep societal cleavages based on religious affiliation. These cleavages have contributed greatly to producing what Barakat (1973) refers to as a "mosaic" society in Lebanon. Each of the religious sects in Lebanon sees itself as distinctly different from the other sects and strives to maintain its autonomy and identity. These aims are facilitated by the development of parallel, but separate, legal and social institutions. For example, according to law as well as tradition, each sect has the power to establish and organize its own system of family laws. These courts have the sole authority to decide on such personal status matters as engagement, marriage, divorce, separation, inheritance, adoption, and tutelage. Civil courts dealing with personal status matters do not exist. Consequently, interfaith marriages are extremely rare; nearly all marriages are between members of the same sect.

In addition, the religious sects have control over the education of their children. Within the extremely loose guidelines set down by the Ministry of Education, each group is permitted to establish its own schools and select the educational materials to be used in them. The effect of the prevalence and autonomy of religious as well as foreign schools in Lebanon (British, German, Japanese, American, Italian, and so forth) has been to retard the development of an adequate Lebanese public school system and a unified educational curriculum.

Religious segregation is not limited simply to the educational system; the great majority of voluntary organizations are also run along religious lines. Membership in youth clubs, women's and men's associations, sports clubs, charitable organizations, and cultural groups is based, by and large, on one's religious affiliation.

The societal cleavages among the religious groups are further strengthened by geographic concentration and segregation. Both on a regional and a local basis, the sects tend to live in specific areas within which they have more or less control. For instance, the Maronites are the overwhelming majority in certain areas of Mount Lebanon – for example, in the Zgharta, Kasruwan, and Batrun districts; the Sunnis are the large majority in the Tripoli and Akkar districts and are one of the largest sects in Beirut; and the Shi'as are clearly the dominant group in South Lebanon. In cities and villages, the religious groups also tend to be segregated into separate neighborhood enclaves.

The major faiths in Lebanon also tend to have different role models to which they refer. The Christians, especially the Maronites, generally closely identify themselves with Western nations (principally France), whereas the Muslims refer to neighboring Arab nations. The Christians rely to a much greater extent on the French language and Western dress and social habits than do the Muslims. Although the Lebanese Muslims stress their Arab heritage, many Christians, particularly the Maronites, prefer to emphasize the distinctiveness of their Phoenician/Mediterranean ancestry.

A further feature of Lebanese society that also runs remarkably well (although not strictly) along religious lines is the presence of significant social, economic, and demographic differentials. Although accurate figures for past and present populations are lacking, it is widely believed that the Christian sects are wealthier, more educated, better clothed and housed, and in more prestigious occupations than the Muslim groups. A good indication of the magnitude of these differentials may be gained from examining the differences among the five religious groups under investigation. We begin by considering religious differentials in the marital characteristics of the groups.

The mean age at marriage for Muslim wives is significantly lower than the figure for Christian wives. Whereas the Christian groups have an average age at marriage of about 21 years, the corresponding average for Muslims falls between 19 and 20 years (19.2 for Sunnis, 19.3 for Shi'as, and 19.9 years for Druzes).[10] Despite this difference in age at first marriage, the average length of marriage duration does not differ significantly among the groups in our sample. This results from the younger age structure of the three Muslim groups. Wife's average age for these three groups is approximately 32.8 years, compared to an average of 34.5 years for Christian wives.

One marital feature that is probably unique to the people in the Middle East is the extent of endogamous marriages, that is, within-family marriages. One-third of the Lebanese couples in the sample were related prior to marriage; half of these couples considered themselves "cousins," and the others stated that they were "distant relatives." As the exact relationships were not ascertained, we are reluctant to place much emphasis on these results. Nevertheless, we do feel that some worthwhile insight might be gained from briefly examining religious differences in the proportion of endogamous marriages. The religious groups with the highest proportions of endogamous marriages are the Druzes and the Shi'as (48 and 46 percent, respectively). The proportions for the Sunnis, Catholics, and non-Catholic Christians are 36, 30, and 22 percent, respectively. Among the two Christian sects the extent of marriage between "cousins" is generally less than half of the endogamous marriages; in contrast, among Muslims the proportion of "cousin" marriages is at least 50 percent. Although endogamous marriages are present among all the religious groups, they are more frequent and more likely to occur between cousins in the Muslim sects.

With such high levels of marriage between relatives, it is not too surprising also to find low rates of intermarriage between the major faiths as well as between sects within them. For the Muslims, marriage between persons from differing Muslim sects is quite unusual. For example, roughly 6 percent of the Sunni males and females had married Shi'as or Druzes. The corresponding proportions for Shi'as and Druzes are even smaller. The proportions of intermarriage between the two Christian groups are substantially greater, ranging from 10 to 20 percent with the non-Catholic Christians having the higher rates. Interfaith marriages are negligible in number in Lebanon; only about 1 percent of the couples had married outside their faith.

As was briefly mentioned earlier, it has historically been the case that the religious groups have occupied certain, well-defined geographic areas – for example, the Maronites and Druzes in Mount Lebanon, the Shi'as in the south, and the Sunnis in the north and in Beirut. The results of the *NFFP* survey are generally in agreement with these patterns. For example, the percentage of all Catholics (mainly Maronites) who are located in Mount Lebanon and Beirut is 38 and 37 percent, respectively. Catholics are considerably fewer in the north and in the Bekaa, and are negligible in the south. Also, although a large proportion of the Catholics live in cities with populations above 10,000, most (55 percent) live in places with populations less than 10,000. The historically based, spatial pattern is also quite evident in the case of Sunnis. The majority of them (55 percent) reside in Beirut; another 33 percent live in the north. The Sunnis are predominantly in the large cities; 84 percent of them live in places with populations of 10,000 and above. A characteristic common to all the religious communities, however, is the attraction to Beirut and its suburbs. A substantial minority of all the groups and a majority of Sunnis reside in Beirut and its suburbs.

No doubt the most pronounced and pervasive differences between the religious communities are socioeconomic in nature. With whatever reasonable criterion one wishes to employ – for example, education, occupation, female labor force participation, income, movie attendance, membership in associations – the socioeconomic differentials that emerge between the religious groups are unmistakably clear: Non-Catholic Christians and Catholics are at the top of the socioeconomic scale, Druzes around the middle, Sunnis near the bottom, and Shi'as at the very bottom. These differences are indicated in Table 3, which examines the educational statuses of the husband and wife, income, husband's occupation, and wife's labor force participation.

The average number of years of schooling completed by non-Catholic Christian, Catholic, and Druze wives is 5.2, 4.4, and 4.5, respectively; all are above the national average of 3.6 years. The Sunni average of 3.3 years is substantially lower. Even lower than the Sunni figure is the average for the Shi'a wives, 1.6 years. The proportion of Shi'a wives with no schooling is 70 percent, nearly twice the national average of 40 percent. A similar pattern exists with respect to husband's education except that the percentage with no schooling among the Druzes is lower than the corresponding percentages for the two Christian groups.

Comparison of the income levels of the groups leads to the same picture that was observed for husband's education. The wealthier groups are the Catholics and the non-Catholics; their average family incomes are 7,173 and 7,112 Lebanese pounds, respectively. The corresponding figures for the Druzes, Sunnis, and Shi'as are 6,180, 5,571, and 4,532 pounds, respectively. (In 1971, one U.S. dollar was roughly equal to three Lebanese pounds.)

Differences in the husband's occupation distributions of the religious groups, although more difficult to compare than income differences, indicate that the Christian husbands are more likely than the husbands of the other groups to be found in the more prestigious, well-paying occupations, and less likely to be employed in low-status, low-income jobs. For instance, consider the proportions who are in the professional/technical versus labor categories: Shi'as, 2 percent versus 35 percent; Sunnis, 4 percent versus 23 percent; Druzes, 3 percent versus 20 percent; Catholics, 6 percent versus 18 percent; and non-Catholic Christians, 6 percent versus 16 percent.

Female labor force participation is also higher among the Christians. Whereas about 28 percent of the Christian wives had worked before marriage, only about 15 percent of the Sunni and Shi'a wives had

Table 3. *Educational status of wife and husband, average family income, husband's occupation, and wife's work experience before and after marriage, by religion: Lebanon, 1971*

Characteristics	Religion					Total
	Catholic	Non-Catholic Christian	Sunni	Shi'a	Druze	
Wife's education						
Average number of years completed	4.4	5.2	3.3	1.6	4.5	3.6
Percentage with no schooling	29%	20%	49%	70%	23%	40%
Husband's education						
Average number of years completed	5.4	5.8	4.5	3.3	5.1	4.9
Percentage with no schooling	15%	13%	29%	31%	10%	21%
Average family income[a]	7,173	7,112	5,571	4,532	6,180	6,247
Percentage with less than 1,500 LL per annum	6%	8%	15%	22%	11%	12%
Husband's occupation						
Professional/technical	6	6	4	2	3	5
Business/managerial	17	21	16	13	20	17
Clerical	14	13	14	10	11	13
Army/police/guard	9	5	5	5	7	6
Crafts/operatives	20	24	22	15	27	21
Farming	10	8	7	11	8	9
Peddlery	0	1	3	4	1	1
Labor	18	16	23	35	20	22
Other	6	7	6	5	4	6
Total	100	100	100	100	100	100
Proportion of wives who worked						
Before marriage	28	27	15	14	22	22
After marriage	10	10	8	6	13	9

[a] In 1971 one U.S. dollar was equal to three Lebanese pounds (LL).

worked. A similar, but less marked, pattern is also observed for labor force participation after marriage. The only exception, however, is the position of the Druze wives. They are somewhat more likely to work after marriage than are Christian wives.

The picture that emerges is one of substantial differentiation along social and economic dimensions between the major faiths as well as considerable differentiation among the Islamic sects. The Muslims are significantly more disadvantaged than the Christians. In addition, although the variation in the characteristics between the two Christian groups is small, the social and economic differences among the Muslim sects are great. The position of the Druzes is clearly superior to that of the Sunnis or Shi'as. The educational levels of the Druze men and women are comparable to those of the Christians. Their annual incomes, although about 1,000 Lebanese pounds less than the average annual incomes of the Christians, are significantly greater than the incomes of the Shi'as or Sunnis. The status of the Sunnis is also superior to that of the Shi'as. The differences between the Sunnis and Shi'as are approximately of the same magnitude as the differences between the Druzes and Sunnis. Shi'as, unequivocally, occupy the lowest social and economic positions of the five major religious groups.

Religious positions on procreation and fertility control

In our investigation of the positions of the religious groups on procreation and fertility control, we differentiated between the official religious doctrines of a sect or group and its particular local orientation. Our main reason for this distinction has been aptly stated by R. A. Fisher:

> It would, I believe, be a fundamental mistake to imagine that the moral attitude of any religious community is to any important extent deducible from the intellectual conceptions of their theology (however much preachers make it their business so to deduce it), and still more to suppose the official doctrine is not itself largely moulded by the state of the popular conscience. (Fisher 1958, p. 222)

It is likely that a religious sect may maintain an official position on fertility control or procreation that is quite different from the attitudes and practices existing among its followers or clergy. For example, Yaukey found that in Lebanon the official religious positions were of little help in explaining religious fertility differentials. In a case where the official doctrine was quite explicit (that is, the Catholic proscription of the use of contraceptives), he found no apparent relation between the proscription and the actual behavior of the sect. Therefore, in the following discussion, we intend first to state the official positions of the religious groups toward procreation and fertility, and then to indicate their local orientations on these subjects.

The official position of the Catholic church is explicit and unambiguous (Noonan 1965; Valsecchi, 1968). With respect to fertility control, the use of chemical or physical contraceptive methods and induced abortion are strictly forbidden. Rhythm is the only method that has been sanctioned by the Catholic church, and may be used only under special circumstances. With regard to procreation, the Catholic church has stressed at various times the value of large families: "Large families are most blest by God and especially loved and prized by the Church as its most precious treasures . . . Large families are the most splendid flowerbeds of the Church" (Pius XII 1958, pp. 363–4).

The position of the other Christian group, the non-Catholic Christians, is less explicit. The Greek Orthodox and Armenian Orthodox (who make up about 90 percent of this group) do not categorically forbid the use of contraception, as do the Catholics. However, they do discourage its use. For example, consider the following remarks concerning the position of the Greek Orthodox: "Though birth control is not mentioned in the binding ecumenical councils, it has been repeatedly disapproved by Orthodox synodical and partriarchal pronouncements and encyclicals. The question of birth control is on the agenda for discussion at a Pan-Orthodox Synod to be held in the future" (Rosten 1975, p. 125). Although these groups are opposed to abortion, they offer tacit approval when medical opinion indicates that the life of the mother is threatened. Procreation is also stressed by these two groups, but not as enthusiastically as by the Catholics.

In contrast to the Christian stances, particularly that of the Catholics, the position of Islam toward procreation and fertility control is more ambiguous, and consequently more open to local and individual interpretation. For example, consider the official view taken at the first international conference on Islam and family planning held in Rabat, Morocco, in December 1971:

> The Islamic Law ensures that the Muslim family will be able to tackle successfully any new situation and have it under control, with correct and sound solutions and measures. That the Islamic Law allows the Muslim family to be able to look after itself as regards the procreation of children, whether this is in the sense of having

many or few of them. It also gives it the right to deal with sterility and to arrange suitably spaced out pregnancies, and to have recourse, when needed to safe and lawful medical means. (Nazer 1974, p. 490)

Such statements have led one scholar to conclude that Islam's "pronatalist position" does not result primarily from its ideology:

> The strong pronatalist orientation of Islam stems less from direct injunctions to procreate than from the support of conditions which make for high fertility. Children are viewed as among the richest blessings granted by Allah, but the Qu'ran also states that good deeds are better than wealth and children; surrender and obedience are the primary values. . . There are references such as "marry and generate" and marry a woman . . . who is richly fruitful," but such references are much less common than in the Torah, for example. (Fagley 1967, p. 83)

Due largely to Islam's structure – for example, the absence of an official religious head, such as the Pope, or a formal governing body – and to its primary reliance on the Koran and Hadiths, each country, religious leader, or scholar is able to render an interpretation of Islam's stance on fertility and control. As a result, numerous differing "official" statements dealing with Islam's position have been made.

The variance in governmental attitudes and activities with respect to the delivery of family planning services also demonstrates the flexibility of Islam (Thorne and Montague 1973). Although some Muslim countries – for example, Egypt, Pakistan, and Tunisia – have active, government-funded family planning programs, others, such as Saudi Arabia and Libyan Arab Jamahiriya, feel that the provision of such services might be in conflict with basic Islamic doctrine.

The position of Islam on induced abortion is also open to interpretation. Although some feel that induced abortion is strictly proscribed, there are others who argue that it is permissible if done before any fetal movement (that is, within the first trimester) or if done to save the mother's life or health. This issue marks a clear distinction among the views of the Shi'as, Sunnis, and Druzes. Although the Shi'as forbid the use of induced abortion at any stage of pregnancy, the Sunnis tend to follow the more liberal position. The Druze position on abortion is less evident. For example, Sheik Halim Taquiyuddin, President of the Druze High Court of Appeal in Lebanon, remarked that abortion for the purposes of birth control is not in principle authorized from a religious standpoint (Nazer 1974, p. 101). However, he did not indicate whether abortion would be permitted by his sect in order to save the life or health of the mother.

In contrast to its positions on procreation, contraception, and abortion, Islam's stand on permanent sterilization is more explicit. According to the 1971 Rabat Conference, sterilization is forbidden: "The Conference considered the question of sterilization and felt that the findings of the Academy of Islamic Research at Al-Azhar are worth following in this matter, namely that the use of means which may lead to sterility is not allowed by the law to the married couple or to anybody else" (Nazer 1974, p. 490).

Having summarized the official positions of the religious groups on procreation and fertility control, we now consider the local orientations of the groups. By local orientations we mean the current attitudes, views, and positions on fertility and fertility control prevailing among the particular religious communities. These local orientations, as noted earlier, are likely to differ considerably from the official laws and doctrines of the religious sects. Probably the best example of how extensive this divergence can be is the substantial difference between the U.S. Catholic community's position on birth control and that of the Vatican (Moore 1973). Another important aspect of local orientation is that it is specific to the religious community of a particular society. For instance, the local orientation of Lebanese Sunnis is most likely different from that of Indonesian or Pakistani Sunnis. Or, in other words, the local orientation of a religious group varies from country to country according to the specifics of the society being considered.

Throughout their histories, Lebanese religious groups have had different affiliations and contacts with outside nations, groups, and cultures – for example, the Maronites with France, the Greek Orthodox with Russia, the Druzes, Jews, and smaller Protestant groups with Britain, and the Sunnis with the Ottomans. By and large, the Christian groups have maintained, and continue to maintain, closer ties with Europe – in particular with France – and with the United States than do the Muslims. The Sunnis and Shi'as, in contrast, have looked more to the Ottoman Empire and neighboring Arab countries. The Druzes have occupied an intermediate position, being neither as Western-oriented as the Christians nor as Arab/Muslim-oriented as the Sunnis and Shi'as.

Migration has also played a key role in differentiating the religious communities. More Lebanese Christians than Lebanese Muslims have migrated to Europe and the Americas (Epstein 1946; Safa 1960; Khuri 1967). Many of these migrants have returned to Lebanon, bringing with them Western thinking, values, and behavior. This differential migratory pattern has made the social and economic differences between the Christians and Muslims even more striking.

Because of the dissimilar affiliations, contacts, and migratory patterns of the religious groups, different role models, values, norms, and aspirations have evolved for Christians, Druzes, and other Muslim groups. The use of contraception and abortion, attitudes toward the structure, function, and size of the family, and the accepted roles for women and children associated with the West seem to have been most readily accepted by the Christians, moderately accepted by the Druzes, and least accepted by the Sunnis and Shi'as.

One indication of the orientations of the religious groups is the attitudes of their members toward fertility control. Irrespective of religious affiliation, the large majority of the Lebanese wives approve of the use of contraception, want to know more about family planning, and disapprove of induced abortion. (Apparently the Lebanese laws forbidding the dispensing of contraceptive materials and information are not in line with the sentiments of most Lebanese couples.)

The ranking, or ordering, of the proportions among the religious groups is not as would be expected from official religious positions. Groups with the strongest sanctions against contraception and abortion have the highest rates of birth control approval among their followers; groups with relatively liberal and flexible positions have followers who are the least approving. For example, the Catholics, the group with the firmest restrictions against contraception and abortion, are among the most approving of these methods. In contrast, the Shi'as, who hold a less restrictive formal position than do the Catholics, express the least favorable attitude toward contraception. These attitudes were discovered by Yaukey (1961), and were also encountered in the WHO (1976) study of Maronites and Shi'as living in the suburbs of Beirut. The World Health Organization found that more Shi'a than Maronite women disapproved of birth control for religious reasons – a finding that is contrary to expectation, as the Roman Catholic church opposes birth control, although Islam does not.

It is reasonably apparent from the histories of the religious groups that the official religious positions do not correspond well to the actual beliefs of the religious communities living in Lebanon. It also seems that reliance on the official positions would mislead us in our attempts to ascertain the extent of pronatalism among the groups and, in turn, to explain religious fertility differentials. Therefore, based on our information and knowledge of the religious groups, we conclude that the two Christian groups are less pronatalist in their positions on procreation and fertility control than are the Muslims, and that among the Muslims, the Druzes are less pronatalist than the Sunnis or Shi'as.

4. Religious fertility differentials

The initial analytical step in this inquiry is to describe the fertility differences among the five major religious groups in Lebanon. This task consists primarily of determining the relative ranking of the groups and the approximate magnitudes of the fertility differences between the groups. The next step is to consider the nature of these religious fertility differentials, that is, to ascertain whether religious affiliation exercises a significant effect on fertility independent of social, economic, and demographic factors – for example, marriage duration, education, income, and residence status.

According to the interaction hypothesis, we should not expect to find the independent variables operating similarly on the fertility of the different religious groups; on the contrary, significant interaction effects should be observed. The relationships of the predictor variables to fertility are expected to differ as a function of the local orientations of the religious groups. For example, education is anticipated to have a greater effect on reducing the fertility of the relatively pronatalist groups (e.g., the Sunnis as opposed to the non-Catholic Christians).

If the interaction terms are minor, that is, if the theory is not correct, then a model stipulating a constant effect of religious affiliation operating across all socioeconomic categories may be utilized to determine the specific effects of religious affiliation on fertility as well as its effect vis-à-vis the other explanatory variables. If, however, the interactions are substantial, then a model that includes interaction terms will be necessary in order to establish properly the effects of religious affiliation on fertility.

In subsequent chapters, similar strategies will be utilized to investigate the probable sources of the religious fertility differentials, namely, differences in the number of children wanted and differences in the willingness and ability to control fertility among the religious groups. Again, the objectives are: (1) to determine the extent of the differences; (2) to decide whether or not there are significant interaction effects; and (3) to develop a model that takes account of these interactions, if they exist, and that specifies the impact of religious affiliation on the dependent variables in relation to the other predictor variables.

Religious fertility differences

In this inquiry into fertility differentials, three measures of fertility are employed: (1) the number of children ever born (NOCEB) per 1,000 married women; (2) the number of living children (NLC) per 1,000 married women; and (3) the proportion of wives who had a live birth in 1970 (LB70), which also yields total fertility rates. Due to differential child survival rates among the religious groups, it is necessary to utilize both NOCEB and NLC.[1] The principal advantage in examining the proportion of wives who had a live birth in 1970 is that it allows current fertility to be considered also.[2]

Contrary to popular thought, there are considerable differences in the number of children ever born and the number of living children among the three Muslim groups (Table 4). At one extreme are the Shi'as. They, by far, have the highest fertility level of any of the religious groups in Lebanon. For example, among wives 40–44 years old, the NOCEB and NLC for Shi'as are 8,247 and 7,290, respectively. At the other extreme are the Druzes; their NOCEB and NLC among wives 40–44 years old are 5,333 and 5,056, respectively. Their fertility level is quite unlike that of the other two Muslim groups; it is much more like the levels found among the Christian groups. Between these extremes are the Sunnis, who, although exhibiting high fertility, have a considerably lower level than the Shi'as. The magnitude of the Muslim fertility differences may be illustrated by the number of living children among wives 40–44 years old. Whereas the Druze women have about five living children, Sunni wives have nearly six, and Shi'as have over seven.

Although the lower fertility levels of the Christian groups may appear similar in comparison to the large Muslim differences, the non-Catholic Christian and Catholic levels are also different from each other. Within each age category, the Catholics have greater numbers of live births and living children than do the non-Catholic Christians. Except for those 45–49 years old, the difference among women near the end of their childbearing careers is half a child or more.

When our measure of current fertility is employed, the preceding conclusions remain unchanged (Table 5). Among Muslims, Shi'as in

Table 4. *Number of children ever born and number of living children per 1,000 married women by religion and wife's age: Lebanon, 1971*

Religion	Wife's age 15–19	20–24	25–29	30–34	35–39	40–44	45–49	All ages	*N*
Number of children ever born per 1,000 married women									
Catholic	632[a]	1,559	2,694	3,878	4,593	5,135	5,200	3,869	925
Non-Catholic Christian	*	1,492	2,266	3,669	4.034	4,223	5,141	3,558	592
Sunni	1,143	2,153	3,963	5,157	6,140	6,358	6,907	4,773	564
Shi'a	1,200	2,557	3,874	5,872	7,098	8,247	8,492	5,714	567
Druze	*	1,263[a]	3,000	4,231	4,950	5,333[a]	*	3,891	119
Total	1,000	1,925	3,147	4,527	5,215	5,900	6,333	4,375	2,767
Number of living children per 1,000 married women									
Catholic	632[a]	1,480	2,625	3,729	4,311	4,771	4,800	3,670	925
Non-Catholic Christian	*	1,476	2,160	3,521	3,729	4,010	4,600	3,328	592
Sunni	1,000	2,031	3,757	4,755	5,570	5,852	5,907	4,365	564
Shi'a	1,150	2,386	3,789	5,456	6,134	7,290	7,222	5,148	566
Druze	*	1,158[a]	2,900	3,962	4,750	5,056[a]	*	3,689	119
Total	944	1,824	3,019	4,277	4,771	5,420	5,598	4,043	2,767

[a] 19 cases in base.

* Less than 20 cases in base.

Table 5. *Proportion of wives who had a live birth in 1970, total fertility rate, and total marital fertility rate by religion and wife's age: Lebanon, 1971*

Religion	15–19	20–24	25–29	30–34	35–39	40–44	45–49	All ages	Total fertility rate	Total marital fertility rate[f]	*N*
Catholic	15.8[a]	34.3	35.0	20.2	11.3	6.5	0.0	17.6	3,808	4,675	925
Non-Catholic Christian	*[b]	40.0	25.5	19.8	6.8	1.9	3.5	15.3	3,325	4,165	592
Sunni	38.0	37.8	35.5	32.4	23.0	7.4	1.9	25.9	5,176	6,670	564
Shi'a	30.0	44.3	46.3	36.0	28.1	17.2	4.8	31.3	6,576	8,165	567
Druze	*[c]	31.6[a]	30.0	15.4	15.0	5.6[a]	*[d]	18.5	3,558	4,920	119
Total	31.0	38.0	35.4	25.8	15.7	7.7	2.2	21.7	4,566	5,690	2,767

[a] Nineteen cases in base.

[b,c,d] In calculating the total fertility rate, proportions *b*, *c*, and *d* were estimated by the following expressions: *b*: (prop. non-Catholic Christian for all ages/prop. Catholic all ages) × (prop. Catholic 15–19); *c*: (prop. Druze for all ages/prop. Catholic all ages) × (prop. Catholic 15–19); *d*: (prop. Catholic 45–49 + prop. non-Catholic Christian)/(2).

[e] In order to calculate the total fertility rates, the national age-specific marital statuses were assumed for each of the five religious groups because age-specific marital statuses for the religious groups are not known.

[f] This is the sum over marriage duration categories for married women.

* Less than 20 cases in base.

virtually every age category have the highest proportion of wives who had live births in 1970; they are followed by Sunnis and then Druzes. The total fertility rates of the three Muslim groups clearly summarize the situation: Shi'a, 6,576; Sunni, 5,176; Druze, 3,558. Among the Christians, we observe that Catholics generally have the higher proportion. The only important change resulting from using current rather than cumulative fertility is the relative position of the Druzes. Whereas Druze cumulative fertility is slightly greater than the Catholic, Druze current fertility is considerably lower than the Catholic rate.

Based on this evidence, two important conclusions seem warranted. First, there are significant fertility differences among Muslim sects and among Christian sects in Lebanon. Therefore, to speak simply of Muslim–Christian fertility differences is misleading. Sect, or denomination, must be taken into account when considering Lebanese religious fertility differentials. Second, the ranking of the groups according to each of the three fertility measures is unequivocal. From high to low fertility the ordering is: Shi'as, Sunnis, Druzes and Catholics (roughly similar), and non-Catholic Christians.

Net effects of religious affiliation

In order to ascertain properly the net effects of religious affiliation on fertility it is necessary to control for the substantial background differences – for example, income, education, and marriage duration – among the religious groups. As there are more than a few characteristics that should be controlled for, the use of contingency tables is limited; consequently, we rely primarily on additive models, employing the multivariate statistical techniques described in Chapter 2, namely, multiple classification analysis (MCA) and dummy variable regression.

Each of the three fertility measures – number of children ever born (NOCEB), number of living children (NLC), and live birth in 1970 (LB70) – is used as a dependent variable in a multiple regression model. The independent variables in the model are: marriage duration (in single years); age at marriage (in single years); wife's education (years of schooling completed); total family income (in Lebanese pounds); size of place of residence (two dummy variables: 10,000 inhabitants or higher; and 1,000 to 9,999 inhabitants, with places with less than 1,000 inhabitants suppressed); religion (four dummy variables: Catholic, Sunni, Shi'a, and Druze, with non-Catholic Christian suppressed).

Other variables, such as district of residence, related premarriage, and wife's work experience before and after marriage, were introduced as controls in these models, but they did not significantly alter the results. Another variable that indicated whether a couple was living in a district in which their religious group was a majority, minority, or neither was added to our regression equation for number of children ever born and number of living children for the entire sample and for each of the religious groups, except the Druzes. The additional variance explained by this variable was not significant and the net effect of minority group status was not consistent among the religious groups. Consequently, we have chosen to omit these variables and to work with the simpler models.

The interaction model differs from the additive model by the inclusion of an interaction: wife's education combined with either Sunni or Shi'a religious affiliation. If the respondent is Sunni or Shi'a, the interaction term will be one times wife's education; otherwise, it will be zero times wife's education, or simply zero.

Interaction terms based on wife's education and on each of the major religious sects were initially entered into the regression models of fertility. The results of these analyses indicated that there were two major clusters: (1) Sunnis and Shi'as, and (2) Catholics, non-Catholic Christians, and Druzes. Subsequent tests of models using the single interaction term, wife's education times Sunni or Shi'a, demonstrated no significant loss in explanatory power over models having interaction terms for each of the religious groups.

The choice of an interaction term employing wife's education was made for several reasons. First, wife's education is a comparatively stable variable, as once obtained, it changes little. Residence status and occupation, for example, are likely to change many times over a ten- to twenty-year period. Residence status is a particularly problematic variable in Lebanon due the the large numbers who at the time of the *NFFP* survey had fled from their rural homes in the south and the Bekaa districts for the relative safety of Beirut and other large urban centers.

Second, of all the variables available for analysis, wife's education is probably the most straightforward and reliable measure of a woman's, or couple's, status. Income was not used because of its questionable reliability as well as because a substantial number of couples (12 percent) did not provide estimates of their income. Husband's occupation was also felt to be less suitable than wife's education due to the extremely broad occupational categories.

Third, inspection of the contingency tables during the preliminary analysis indicated that certain interactions were more probable than others. Fertility differences among the religious sects were found to be greatly reduced as wife's education was increased. For example, for wives who had not completed primary school the number of children ever born per 1,000 married women was 6,612 for Sunnis and 4,938 for non-Catholic Christians, for a difference of 1,674. The numbers of live births for Sunni and non-Catholic Christian wives of the same age but who had completed secondary or higher schooling were 2,545 and 3,037, respectively, for a difference of 492. Not only have the differentials converged, but at higher levels of education the Sunnis actually demonstrate lower fertility than do the non-Catholic Christians.

Turning to results of the dummy variable regressions, we find that the interaction term of wife's education and religious affiliation contributes a significant amount of explanatory power in the case of NOCEB and NLC, but not for LB70. The F ratios for number of children ever born and number of living children are significant at the .001 and .05 levels, respectively. This implies that the interaction model, at least for NOCEB and NLC, is statistically the more appropriate one to utilize. For the proportion who had a live birth in 1970 (LB70), the amount of variance explained by including the interaction term is zero. Therefore, owing to these results, wife's education and religious affiliation, $WE \times R$, are combined into a single variable for the multiple classification analyses (MCA) of NOCEB and NLC; for the third dependent variable, LB70, wife's education and religion are considered separately.

For both NOCEB and NLC, $WE \times R$ has a greater effect on fertility than age at marriage, total family income, husband's occupation, or residence status; marriage duration, as would be expected, has the greatest single effect (Tables A.1 and A.2). Except for marriage duration, $WE \times R$'s gross effect, R^2 (eta squared), and its net effect, R^2 (multiple partial coefficient squared), are substantially larger than any of the other explanatory variables. Moreover, the proportion of variance in NOCEB and NLC explained by $WE \times R$ over and above that explained by marriage duration, total family income, husband's occupation, and residence status is considerable: 13.2 and 10.9 percent, respectively.

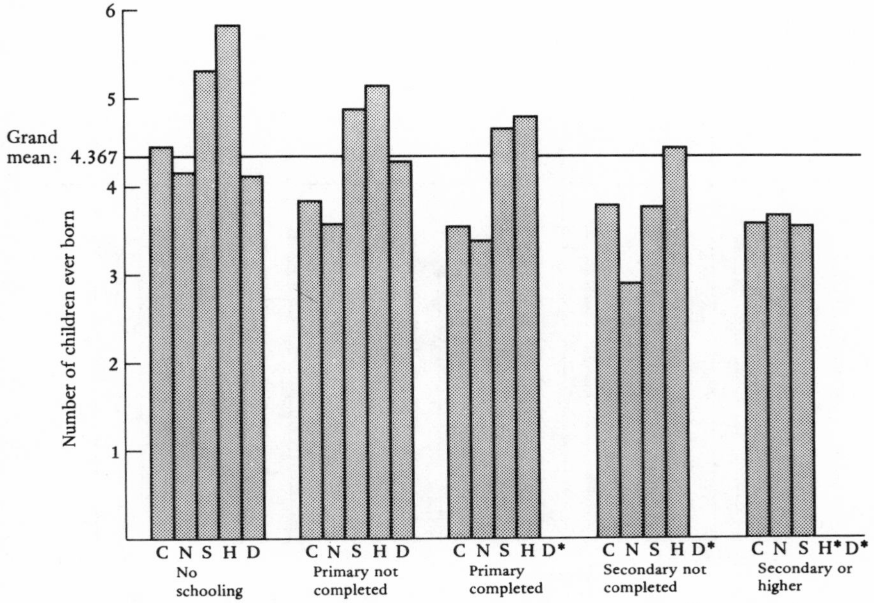

Note: Religion by wife's education (C = Catholic; N = Non-Catholic Christian; S = Sunni; H = Shi'a; D = Druze)
*Less than 20 cases in base

Figure 3. The effect of wife's education on number of children ever born by religious affiliation net of marriage duration, marriage age, income, husband's occupation, and size of place of residence: Lebanon, 1971.

As an aid to the discussion, the pattern of religious fertility differentials is illustrated in Figures 3 and 4. Though several categories have been deleted due to small numbers of cases, the results of these figures are clear: At low levels of education, differences in religious affiliation lead to substantial fertility differentials; at high levels of education, differences in religious affiliation lead to lesser fertility differentials.[3] Among wives with primary education or less, fertility differentials are much the same as were noted earlier in the discussion. Namely, Shi'as show the highest fertility, followed by Sunnis, then by Catholics and Druzes, and finally by non-Catholic Christians. In contrast, among wives with more than primary education, the situation is considerably different. Ignoring Druzes and Shi'as due to their small case numbers, one observes relatively low fertility for Catholics, Sunnis, and non-Catholic Christians, and much smaller fertility differentials than existed between these groups at lower levels of wife's education.

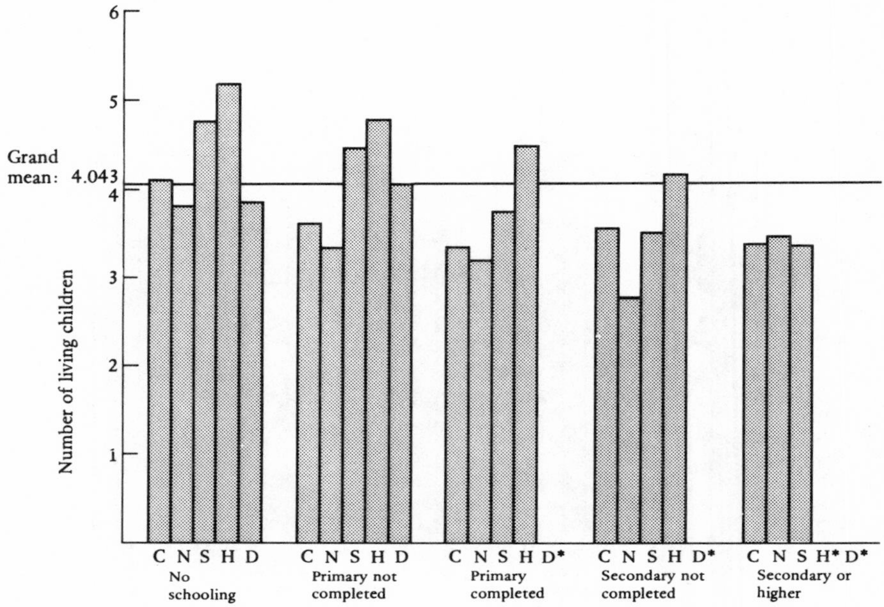

Note: Religion by wife's education (C = Catholic; N = Non-Catholic Christian; S = Sunni; H = Shi'a; D = Druze)
*Less than 20 cases in base

Figure 4. The effect of wife's education on number of living children by religious affiliation net of marriage duration, marriage age, income, husband's occupation, and size of place of residence: Lebanon, 1971.

As a specific example, consider the fertility of Catholics and Sunnis. Among wives with no schooling, the net effect of being a Sunni rather than a Catholic results in having 0.874 more live births and 0.650 more living children. For wives with more than primary education, the net effect of being Sunni rather than Catholic means having virtually the same fertility. In fact, the net effects for Sunnis are slightly less than they are for Catholics.

As dummy variable regression showed that the inclusion of the interaction term, $WE \times R$, does not lead to a significant increase in R^2, religion and wife's education were entered as separate variables in the multiple classification analysis of the third fertility measure, LB70 (Table A.3). After controlling for marriage duration, age at marriage, wife's education, total family income, husband's occupation, and residence status, there continue to be substantial religious differences in the proportion of wives who had a live birth in 1970. When the net effects of religion are added to the grand mean, the following figures are obtained for the proportion of wives who had a live birth in 1970: Shi'as, 29.7; Sunnis, 24.5; Catholics, 18.5; Druzes, 17.7; and non-Catholic Christians, 17.1. This ranking is similar to the one based on cumulative fertility for wives with low levels of education.

The relative importance of religion as an explanatory variable for LB70 is high. After marriage duration, religion has the largest proportion of explained variance. Its eta squared and multiple partial coefficient squared are 2.2 and 1.2 percent, respectively, which are considerably greater than the corresponding figures for wife's education, 0.4 and 0.2 percent, respectively.

At this point one may ask why the third measure of fertility, the proportion who had a live birth in 1970 (LB70), yields results that are different from the other two measures of fertility. There are several reasons for this discrepancy. First, the mix of factors that influence having a live birth in a particular year is likely not to be the same as the one that affects cumulative fertility. Wife's education, residence status, income, and so forth, may have relatively small effects (as compared to characteristics such as age, marriage duration, and parity) on whether a woman has a live birth in a given year. An interaction term is likely to have an even smaller effect.

Another possible cause for the discrepancy is statistical in nature. When a dependent variable is a dichotomy, certain problems arise in using ordinary least squares methods (see Goldberger 1964; Goodman 1973; and Nerlove and Press 1973 for a full discussion). These problems are especially severe when the split on the dichotomous variable is quite unbalanced, that is, when the mean falls outside the range of 0.2 to 0.8. As the grand mean for LB70 is 0.217, the results of dummy variable regression and MCA for this variable should be viewed with greater caution and skepticism than the results obtained from the other two fertility measures.

In general, then, the results of the multivariate analyses for cumulative fertility tend to be consistent with the interaction hypothesis. That is, religious fertility differentials are dependent on the levels of the social and economic statuses of the religious groups being considered, with the groups near the ends of the scale having basically similar fertility, but with evident differences for those located in the middle portion of the scale. However, except for societies with a high degree of socioeconomic diversity, the entire pattern of religious fertility differentials is unlikely to be encountered with data taken at a single point in time. Apparently this appears to be the case in our inquiry. Although limited in its representation of socioeconomic statuses, the investigation of the Lebanese data produces a pattern represented by the right-hand half of Figure 2.

Further discussion and interpretation of the findings in relation to the interaction hypothesis are in order. However, it is preferable first to complete the empirical portion of our investigation by examining religious differences with respect to family size preferences, and religious differences regarding family planning knowledge, attitudes, and practices. Analyses of these differences will provide a more thorough understanding of religious fertility differentials as well as enrich the interpretation and discussion of the findings vis-à-vis the interaction hypothesis.

5. Religious differentials in family size preferences

Differences in ideal number of children and additional number wanted

The respondents considered four children, on the average, to be the ideal family size. The ideals of the five religious groups fall within a one-child range around this mean (Table 6). Surprisingly, the lowest ideal number of children preferred, one-half less than the national average, exists among the Druze wives. The non-Catholic Christians were second lowest, followed closely by Sunnis and Catholics, who wanted the same average number of children. The highest ideal number of children (4.5) was expressed by the Shi'as.

When controlling for parity, the effect of wife's age on the ideal number of children appears minimal (Table 6). Parity, in contrast, has a strong impact on ideals. For each of the religious groups, we find that the higher the parity of a woman, the greater her ideal number of children. For example, those of parity one stated ideals approximately one child less than wives at parity six and higher. The introduction of these controls, however, does not greatly alter the basic relationship existing among the religious groups. Shi'as continue to express the largest ideal number of children, whereas Druzes have the lowest ideals; between the Shi'as and the Druzes fall the ideals of the non-Catholics, Sunnis, and Catholics, with the Sunnis usually having a slightly lower ideal number than the Catholics.

Irrespective of ideal number of children, or current parity, each of the religious groups maintains a clear preference for sons. The sex ratios of ideal number of sons to ideal number of daughters generally range from 1.20 to 1.40. The only exception to this pattern is when the ideal number of children is two or four. In these instances, the sex ratios are all less than 1.20, with most falling between 1.04 and 1.10.

The ranking of the religious groups in terms of these sex ratios is similar to the one noted for ideal number of children. The sex prefer-

Table 6. *Ideal number of children reported by religion, wife's age, and parity: Lebanon, 1971*

Wife's age and parity	Religion Catholic	Non-Catholic Christian	Sunni	Shi'a	Druze	Total
15–29						
0–1	3.3	3.3	3.5	3.9	*	3.4
2–4	3.7	3.7	3.7	4.1	3.4	3.8
5+	*	*	4.3	4.4	*	4.4
30–39						
0–1	3.4	*	*	*	*	3.3
2–4	3.7	3.5	3.5	3.8	*	3.5
5+	4.5	4.3	4.2	5.1	3.8	4.5
40–49						
0–1	*	*	*	*	*	3.5
2–4	4.0	3.6	3.8	*	3.8[a]	3.8
5+	4.7	4.3	4.4	4.9		4.5
All wives	3.9	3.7	3.9	4.5	3.5	4.0
N	730	486	415	391	99	2,121

[a]Number refers to the two-and-above parity category.

*Less than 20 cases in base.

ence ratios for Druzes and non-Catholic Christians are the lowest, followed by those for Sunnis and Catholics; the highest ratios are among the Shi'a wives.

The second measure with which we intend to investigate religious differences in family size norms is the number of additional children wanted. The percent wanting additional children by religious affiliation, wife's age, and number of living children is shown in Table 7. The overall picture is very similar to that observed earlier in the case of ideal numbers of children. For most age and parity levels, the proportion wanting additional children is smallest among the Druzes and non-Catholic Christians; Catholics and Sunnis have somewhat higher percentages; and Shi'as have the largest proportion. As an illustration of this pattern consider the percentages wanting additional children among wives aged 30–39 with two to four children: Druzes, 21; non-Catholic Christians, 34; Sunnis, 41; Catholics 44; Shi'as, 61.

In addition, at each parity level, the Shi'as wanted substantially more children than any of the other religious sects. At parity three, for

Table 7. *Percentage of wives wanting additional children by religion, wife's age, and number of living children: Lebanon, 1971*

Wife's age and number of living children	Religion: Catholic	Non-Catholic Christian	Sunni	Shi'a	Druze	Total
15–29						
0–1	89	93	97	98	*	94
2–4	59	57	61	72	59	62
5+	22	*	44	35	*	37
30–39						
0–1	79	*	*	*	*	90
2–4	44	34	41	61	21	41
5+	24	15	19	39	*	23
40–49						
0–1	*	*	*	*	*	66
2–4	15	11	21	*	7[a]	15
All wives	41	40	37	43	41	40
N	925	592	564	566	119	2,766

[a] Refers to the two-and-above parity category.
*Less than 20 cases in base.

example, the Shi'as wanted about one and a half additional children. In contrast, the other religious groups wanted, on the average, an additional one-half child. In general, non-Catholic Christians wanted the smallest numbers of additional children. By parity four, nearly all of the non-Catholic Christians wives wanted no further children. The numbers desired by the Catholics and Sunnis were nearly the same, with the Sunnis wanting slightly more. For example, of the Sunni and Catholic wives who had had four live births, approximately one out of every three wives wanted an additional child.

Net effects of religious affiliation on family size preferences

Up to this point, the discussion has rested on controls for wife's age and parity. The next issue to be addressed is whether or not the findings will remain unchanged with the introduction of further controls such as husband's occupation, family income, wife's education, and residence status.

The additive model in the dummy variable regressions consists of seven major independent variables: (1) marriage duration; (2) age at marriage; (3) parity; (4) wife's education; (5) total family income; (6) size of place of residence (two dummy variables: 10,000 inhabitants or higher; and 1,000 to 9,999 inhabitants, with places with less than 1,000 inhabitants suppressed); (7) religion (four dummy variables: Catholic, non-Catholic Christian, Sunni, and Druze, with Shi'a suppressed). Again, the interaction model differs from the additive one by a single term: wife's education combined with Sunni or Shi'a religious affiliation. Given the importance of wife's education in determining family size preferences, it is believed that if this interaction were found to be insignificant, then the likelihood of others being significant would be small.

The results of the dummy variable regressions indicate that the models with the interaction term do not yield significant improvements over the simpler additive models. Neither of the F ratios is significant, indicating no statistical justification for the inclusion of the interaction term. The relationship between wife's education and the two dependent variables may therefore be assumed to be the same for the five religious groups.

Although one may work with the results of dummy variable regression to ascertain the differences in family size preferences among the religious groups, we again choose to utilize results from multiple classification analysis (MCA). The reason for this choice is that the results produced by MCA are felt to be in a somewhat more convenient form for our purposes.

The net effect of religion on ideal number of children (1.5 percent) is not very different from the net effects of wife's education, husband's occupation, and residence size (Table A.4). Parity has a substantially larger net effect than religion (2.4 percent versus 1.5 percent). Marriage duration and age at marriage, as might be expected from our earlier findings concerning the effect of wife's age on ideal number of children, have negligible net effects.

After controlling for marriage duration, age at marriage, parity, wife's education, income, husband's occupation, and residence, the effects of religious affiliation on ideal number of children are reduced for all of the religious groups except the Druzes. For example, the gross effect of being a non-Catholic Christian is −0.300; after controls have been applied, the effect is −0.143. In other words, their ideal number of children increases from 3.674 to 3.831. Except for differentials involving Druzes, the differences among the religious groups in ideal number of children are attenuated when the influences of differing background characteristics are removed.

Despite these controls, however, the relative ranking of ideal number of children among the religious groups remains unchanged: Druzes, 3.4 children; non-Catholic Christians, 3.8; Sunnis, 3.9; Catholics, 3.9; Shi'as, 4.4. The introduction of further controls beyond wife's age and parity does not significantly alter our earlier conclusions concerning religious differences in ideal number of children. On the contrary, the results of these regression analyses strengthen our confidence in those conclusions.

In contrast to its effect on ideal number of children, after parity and marriage duration, religion has the largest net effect (2.2 percent) on the number of additional children wanted (Table A.5). Age at marriage, wife's education, husband's occupation, total family income, and size of place of residence all have relatively minor effects. Their multiple partial coefficients are 0.5 percent or less.

The net effects of religion on the number of additional children wanted yield differentials that, on the whole, are consistent with the findings found when controlling for parity only. Shi'as desire substantially more additional children than any of the other religious groups. Non-Catholic Christians, on the other hand, want the smallest number of additional children. They are followed by Druzes, Catholics, and Sunnis, in that order. Although there are differences among these last four groups, these differences are relatively minor in relation to comparisons involving Shi'as.

6. Religious differentials in fertility control knowledge, attitudes, and practices

Knowledge

Religious differences in knowledge of fertility control methods were not fixed; the groups varied considerably by birth control technique (Table 8). Catholics and non-Catholic Christians were more knowledgeable about coitus interruptus, the condom, and rhythm than were the other sects. The Sunnis and Shi'as were more knowledgeable with respect to tubal ligation, the cervical cap, and (to a lesser extent) the IUD. The five sects were about equally knowledgeable about several other methods, such as the oral pill and the sponge.

In general, however, despite the few exceptions, such as the oral pill, these differences suggest a "conventional-modern" division in knowledge of contraception among the four largest sects. It appears that the two Christian groups are more familiar with traditional techniques, whereas the Sunnis and the Shi'as, although to a lesser extent, are more aware of modern methods.

Given that there are twelve different birth control methods, it would be impractical to consider the net effect of religious affiliation on each of these techniques. Consequently, we have chosen to investigate two contraceptive techniques, one traditional, coitus interruptus, and one modern, tubal ligation. The proportions of women having knowledge of coitus interruptus and tubal ligation were selected on the basis of preliminary analyses which suggested substantial variation in knowledge of these methods among the religious groups.

According to the results of dummy variable regression, a model employing an interaction term for wife's education and religion was found to be statistically more appropriate than a simple, additive model. Consequently, wife's education and religion are considered as a single predictor ($WE \times R$) in the MCA analysis.

The MCA analysis of familiarity with coitus interruptus consists of seven predictors: (1) marriage duration; (2) age at marriage; (3) parity;

Table 8. *Proportion of wives having knowledge of various contraceptive methods by religion: Lebanon, 1971*

	Religion					
Method	Catholic	Non-Catholic Christian	Sunni	Shi'a	Druze	Total
Coitus interruptus	89	90	79	55	82	80
Condom	80	81	76	62	66	75
Rhythm	62	65	53	35	46	54
Douche	51	59	56	37	50	51
Sponge	13	9	14	10	5	11
Vaginal tablet	49	52	56	34	42	48
Cream	10	10	8	6	11	9
Cervical cap	24	25	56	34	42	48
Oral pill	90	96	90	90	90	91
Tubal ligation	40	39	47	51	34	43
IUD	23	24	37	22	24	26
Vasectomy	10	10	13	9	10	11
N	925	592	564	567	119	2,767

(4) wife's education × religion; (5) total family income; (6) husband's occupation; and (7) size of place of residence (Table A.6). The predictor with the largest gross and net effects is wife's education × religion (14 and 11 percent, respectively). Its effects are substantially greater than those of any of the other variables. Size of place of residence is the only other variable that has a notable impact on familiarity with coitus interruptus (4 and 3 percent, respectively). The larger the size of the place of residence, the greater the proportion of women familiar with coitus interruptus. The net effects of marriage duration, parity, and age at marriage are small; the combined net effect of these three variables is approximately 0.5 percent. The net effects of total family incomes and husband's occupation (0.2 and 1.6 percent, respectively) are also small in comparison to the effects of *WE* × *R* and residence status.

The net effects of wife's education and religious affiliation are illustrated in Figure 5. This figure prompts at least two significant conclusions. First, the net effect of wife's education varies according to religious affiliation. For Catholics and non-Catholic Christians, and

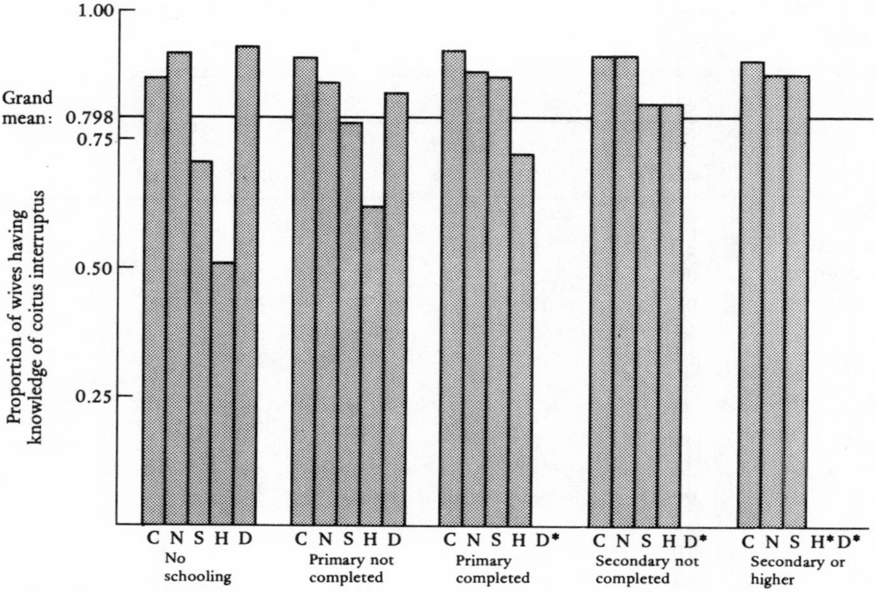

Note: Religion by wife's education (C = Catholic; N = Non-Catholic Christian; S = Sunni; H = Shi'a; D = Druze)
*Less than 20 cases in base

Figure 5. The effect of wife's education on the proportion of wives having knowledge of coitus interruptus by religious affiliation net of marriage duration, marriage age, parity, income, husband's occupation, and size of place of residence: Lebanon, 1971.

perhaps for Druzes, the net effect of wife's education is minimal and irregular. For example, the variation in knowledge of coitus interruptus is less than 5 percent for Catholic wives. In contrast, the net effect of wife's education is sizable for Shi'as and Sunnis. Generally, the higher the level of education, the larger the proportion aware of coitus interruptus. Among Shi'as, for example, the proportion varies from 51 percent for wives with no schooling to 82 percent for those who did not complete secondary school.

Second, religious differences in the proportion aware of coitus interruptus diminish to insignificance with increased education. Whereas at low levels of education the differences between the Christian sects versus the Sunnis and Shi'as are great, the differences are small or nonexistent at higher levels of education. This convergence is most apparent in the case of Sunnis and non-Catholic Christians. At the lowest levels of wife's education, the proportion aware of coitus interruptus is 93 percent for non-Catholic Christians and 71 percent for Sunnis, for a difference of 22 percent. Among wives who completed secondary school or higher, the proportion is 87 percent for both non-Catholic Christians and Sunnis.

In contrast to knowledge about coitus interruptus, the proportion familiar with tubal ligation is significantly greater among Shi'as and Sunnis: Shi'as, 51 percent; Sunnis, 47 percent; Catholics, 40 percent; non-Catholic Christians, 39 percent; and Druzes, 34 percent. The introduction of controls for differences in background characteristics in no way reduces the substantially higher positions of Shi'as and Sunnis. On the contrary, although our dummy variable regression results indicate a significant interaction between religion, wife's education, and the proportion having knowledge of tubal ligation, the differences in the proportions among the groups do *not* converge with increases in wife's education, as was the case for coitus interruptus; rather, they diverge.

This divergence is clearly evidenced by our MCA results (Table A.7 and Figure 6). For wives with no schooling, the largest difference in the net proportions familiar with tubal ligation, 18 percent, exists between the Shi'as and the non-Catholic Christians (48 and 30 percent, respectively). The difference increases to 32 percent when Shi'a and non-Catholic wives who had not completed secondary school are considered (76 and 44 percent, respectively).

As in the case of coitus interruptus, wife's education × religion (*WE* × *R*) has the largest effect on familiarity with tubal ligation; however, in comparison to the other predictors, its relative effect is smaller than it was for coitus interruptus. The gross and net effects of *WE* × *R* are 8 and 3 percent, respectively. The second most important variable is residence size; its gross and net effects are 5 and 2 percent, respectively. Again, as was found with coitus interruptus, the larger the place of residence, the greater is the proportion of women familiar with tubal ligation.

Marriage duration, age at marriage, and parity have negligible effects on familiarity with tubal ligation. Their combined net effect is no greater than 0.5 percent. The effects of total family income and husband's occupation are somewhat greater (1 to 2 percent). In general, couples who had higher-status occupations and higher incomes were more likely to be familiar with tubal ligation.

In sum, the picture that emerges is not simply one of Catholics and non-Catholic Christians having greater knowledge of fertility control

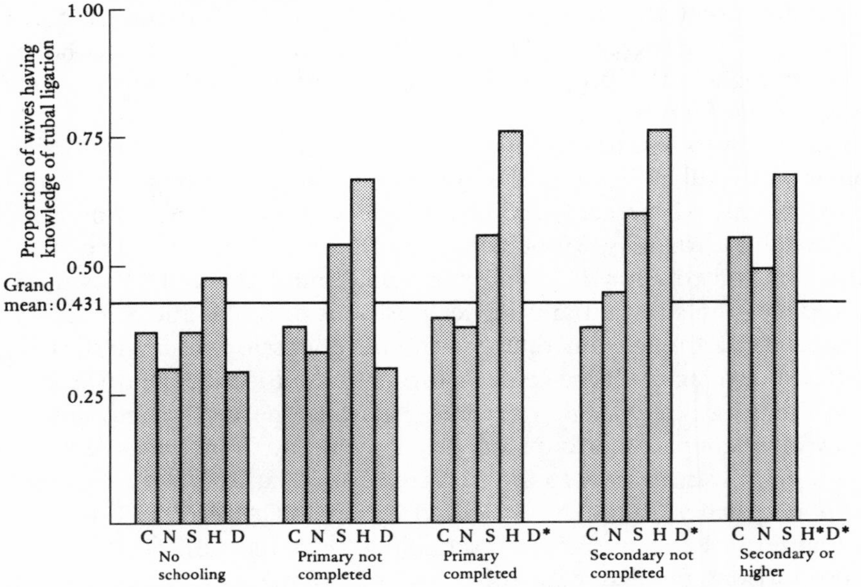

Note: Religion by wife's education (C = Catholic; N = Non-Catholic Christian; S = Sunni; H = Shi'a; D = Druze)
*Less than 20 cases in base

Figure 6. The effect of wife's education on the proportion of wives having knowledge of tubal ligation by religious affiliation net of marriage duration, marriage age, parity, income, husband's occupation, and size of place of residence: Lebanon, 1971.

than Sunnis, Shi'as, or Druzes. The situation is more complex because the conclusions depend not only on the particular measure of knowledge utilized, but also on the level of wife's education considered. Consequently, the answer to the issue of religious differences in knowledge of fertility control has several aspects: (1) Among illiterate and poorly educated couples, the two Christian sects are more knowledgeable about coitus interruptus (and probably other traditional methods) than are the Muslim groups; however, these differences are substantially less at higher levels of education, and among wives who completed secondary school or higher, the differences are minor; and (2) regardless of the level of wife's education, Sunnis and Shi'as are more familiar with tubal ligation than are Catholics, non-Catholic Christians, and Druzes.

Attitudes

To ascertain the extent of religious differences in attitudes toward fertility control, two measures were utilized: (1) wife's approval of contraceptive use and (2) wife's desire for additional information about family planning. In general, contraceptive use is approved of by Lebanese wives. Three out of every four wives between the ages of 15 and 49 years approved of its use. Except for Shi'a wives, approval of contraceptive use did not differ greatly among the religious groups: (1) Druzes, 82 percent; (2) Catholics, 77 percent; (3) non-Catholic Christians, 76 percent; (4) Sunnis, 76 percent; and (5) Shi'as, 56 percent.

The ranking of the religious groups according to approval of contraceptive use is not substantially modified when wife's age and number of living children are considered. The Druzes and Shi'as remain at the high and low extremes, respectively, whereas the Catholics, non-Catholic Christians, and Sunnis fall in between, with no fixed ranking among them.

Approximately two-thirds of the wives stated a desire for further information about family planning. The religious sect least desiring further information was the Shi'a (58 percent). The other four groups were similar to each other in their desire for further information (68 to 73 percent). It should be noted that among these four groups, the Christian sects were not, as is sometimes believed, the most interested in receiving additional information on family planning. Sunni wives represented the highest proportion, 73 percent, and close behind them were the Druzes and non-Catholic Christians with 71 percent each. Controls for wife's age and number of living children, in most instances, did not greatly affect the relative ranking of the groups.

To gain further insight into the religious differences in attitudes toward fertility control, dummy variable regression and MCA were again relied upon. Given the interactive patterns encountered earlier, an interaction among religion, wife's education, and attitude toward contraceptive use was anticipated. Dummy variable regression confirmed that this interaction was significant.

Among the seven independent variables used in the MCA analysis of the proportion of wives who approved of contraceptive use, wife's education × religion had the largest net effect, 3.4 percent (Table A.8). Size of place of residence and husband's occupation also had large net effects, 2.7 and 2.2 percent, respectively. The pattern of net effects for these two variables was generally as would be expected. For instance, approval of contraceptive use was positively related to size of place of residence: (1) 78 percent for places with 10,000 or more inhabitants; (2) 73 percent for places with 1,000 to 9,999 inhabitants; and (3) 63 percent for places with less than 1,000 inhabitants.

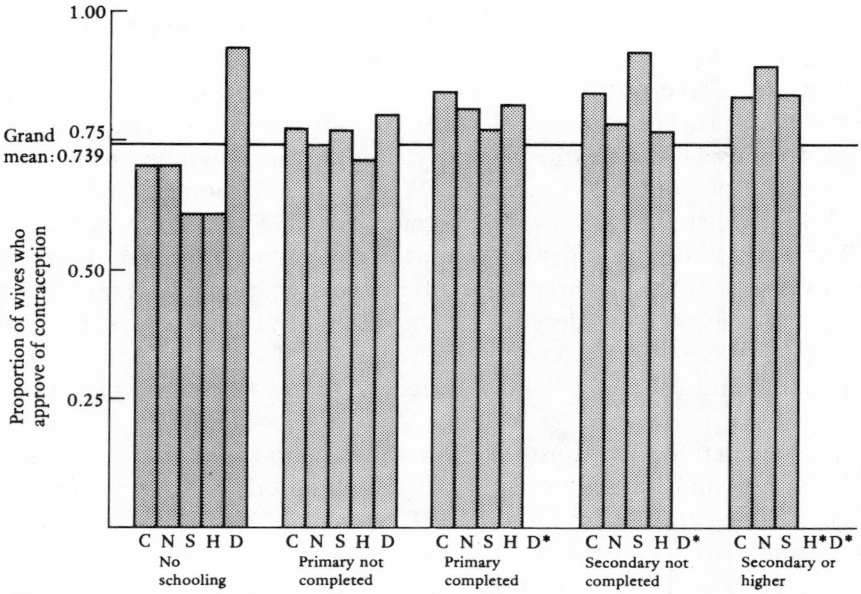

Note: Religion by wife's education (C = Catholic; N = Non-Catholic Christian; S = Sunni, H = Shi'a; D = Druze)
*Less than 20 cases in base

Figure 7. The effect of wife's education on the proportion of wives who approve of contraception by religious affiliation net of marriage duration, marriage age, parity, income, husband's occupation, and size of place of residence: Lebanon, 1971.

The net effects for the religious groups according to wife's educational level are illustrated in Figure 7. The effect of wife's education is reasonably clear and similar among each of the religious groups (except the Druzes, whose numbers are too small for comparisons). That is, the proportion approving of contraceptive use increases as wife's education increases.

In contrast, the pattern of the religious differences is less apparent. In some cases the differences converge (non-Catholic Christian versus Shi'a), and in others they diverge (non-Catholic Christian versus Sunni). What seems clear, however, is that the Muslim sects do not have rates that are consistently lower than the Christian groups. Only at the level of no schooling do the Sunnis and Shi'as have rates of approval of contraceptive use that are lower than those for the Catholics and non-Catholic Christians. At the other four educational levels, the proportions for the Muslim sects are either similar to or greater than the proportions for the Christian denominations. For example, the proportions among wives who did not complete secondary school but completed primary school are: (1) Sunni, 92 percent; (2) Catholic, 84 percent; (3) non-Catholic Christian, 78 percent; and (4) Shi'a, 76 percent. The commonly heard statements concerning the less favorable attitudes of the Muslims toward contraceptive use are not born out by the data.

Our second measure of attitudes toward fertility control is the proportion of wives who want to know more about family planning. Approximately two-thirds of the wives stated a desire for further information about family planning. The ranking of the religious groups with respect to the desire for family planning information was: Sunnis, 73 percent; Druzes, 71 percent; non-Catholic Christians, 71 percent; Catholics, 68 percent; Shi'as, 58 percent.

Controlling for wife's age, number of living children, and wife's education does little to affect the relative ranking of the groups' desire for family planning information. For each of the religious sects, higher education is related to greater willingness to learn about family planning. However, given the findings from previous sections, a test for interaction was performed. The results of the dummy variable regression indicated that the interaction $WE \times R$ was not statistically significant. Consequently, the simple additive model was selected for the multiple classification analysis of the net effects of religious affiliation on the proportion wanting more information on family planning.

There are at least two major points that may be made on the basis of the MCA results (Table A.9). First, relative to the other independent variables, the influence of religion is not great. The variables that have the largest impact on whether a woman states that she wants more information about family planning are marriage duration and parity; together these variables account for approximately half of the explained variance. The effect of religion is considerably less. Its multiple partial coefficient is about one-fourth of the coefficient for marriage duration and parity (1.4 versus 6.3 percent, respectively). Religion's influence is about the same as age at marriage and residence size, but it is greater than the effects of wife's education, total family income, and husband's occupation.

Second, apart from the low proportion for Shi'as, there is very little difference among the religious groups in their desire for further information about family planning, either on a gross or net effect basis. A substantial majority of every religious group want to know more about family planning, and with some exceptions (namely, those comparisons involving Shi'as), they differ little in this respect.

Practices

Based on the proportions who had ever used contraception and who were currently using contraception at the time of the survey, the religious groups may be divided into three classes of fertility control usage: (1) high: Catholics, non-Catholic Christians, and Druzes, 70–78 percent ever used and 60–62 percent currently using; (2) intermediate: Sunnis, 62 percent ever used and 49 percent currently using; and (3) low: Shi'as, 47 percent ever used and 35 percent currently using. The magnitudes of the religious differentials in past contraceptive use are very similar to the religious differences in current contraceptive use. For instance, between non-Catholic Christians and Shi'as the difference in the proportions who had ever used contraception was 26 percent, compared to a 25 percent difference in the proportions currently contracepting.

Controls for wife's age and number of living children have little effect on the differences in fertility control usage among the religious groups. Except for the 45–49-year-old group, it is generally the case that for each of the religious sects, the proportions who had ever used contraception and who were currently using contraception vary directly with wife's age. Number of living children is also related to past and current contraceptive use in that the proportions are greatest for those with two to four living children and least for those with no children or one child.

We observed earlier that the religious groups seemed to be divided in their knowledge of contraceptive methods. Although there were a few exceptions, the Catholics and non-Catholic Christians appeared to be more familiar with traditional techniques, whereas the Shi'as and particularly the Sunnis were more aware of certain modern methods. Examination of the proportions who had ever used or who were currently using contraception by specific method suggests that there is a similar, although less pronounced, division in the use of contraception (Table 9). Catholics and non-Catholic Christians had used and were currently using coitus interruptus, the condom, and rhythm more extensively than the Sunnis and Shi'as, and the Sunnis and Shi'as had relied upon and were still using to a greater extent the oral pill. For example, the proportion currently using rhythm was 9 percent for Catholics, 9 percent for non-Catholic Christians, 4 percent for Druzes, 4 percent for Sunnis, and 2 percent for Shi'as. In contrast, the proportion who were currently using the oral pill was 20 percent for Sunnis, 17

Table 9. *Proportion of wives who ever used and who are currently using various contraceptive methods by religion: Lebanon, 1971*

	Religion					
Method	Catholic	Non-Catholic Christian	Sunni	Shi'a	Druze	Total
Ever used:						
Coitus interruptus	62	50	37	24	54	56
Condom	28	24	23	15	24	23
Rhythm	22	18	11	6	12	15
Douche	13	14	11	9	15	12
Sponge	1	0	1	1	1	1
Vaginal tablet	8	7	6	3	8	6
Cream	0	1	1	1	1	1
Cervical cap	1	1	1	1	1	1
Oral pill	25	29	34	30	27	30
Tubal ligation	1	1	1	1	1	1
IUD	1	2	1	1	1	1
Vasectomy	0	0	0	0	0	0
Any method	78	73	62	47	71	67
Currently using:						
Coitus interruptus	40	32	20	10	33	27
Condom	10	9	6	4	8	8
Rhythm	9	9	4	2	4	6
Douche	13	14	11	9	15	12
Sponge	0	0	0	0	0	0
Vaginal tablet	2	1	1	0	3	1
Cream	0	1	0	0	0	0
Cervical cap	0	0	0	0	0	0
Oral pill	10	12	20	17	15	14
Tubal ligation	1	1	1	1	1	1
IUD	0	2	1	1	1	1
Vasectomy	0	0	0	0	0	0
Any method	62	60	49	35	60	53
N	925	592	564	567	119	2,767

percent for Shi'as, 15 percent for Druzes, 12 percent for non-Catholic Christians, and 10 percent for Catholics. The use of tubal ligation, the IUD, and vasectomy was low for all the groups. The newness and limited availability of these modern methods may account for the absence of differentials between the two clusters of religious groups.

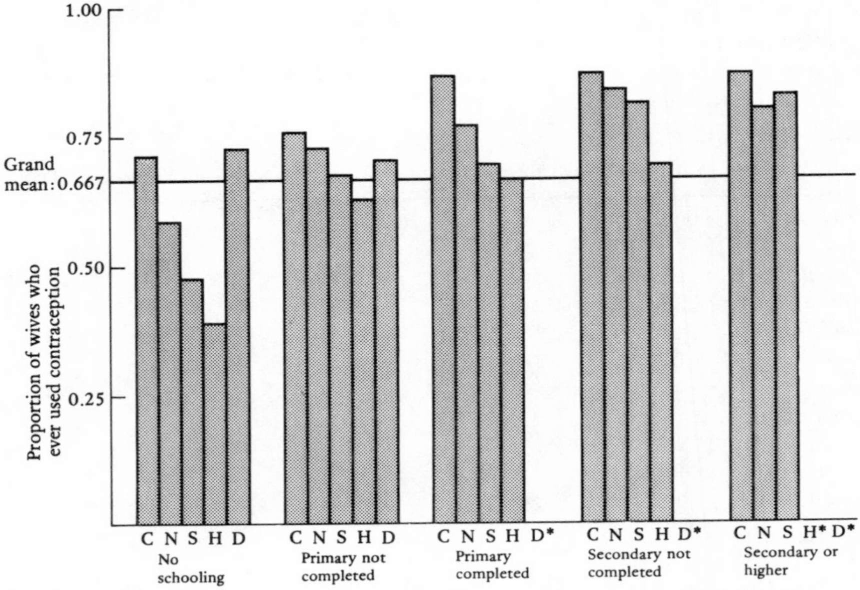

Note: Religion by wife's education (C = Catholic; N = Non-Catholic Christian; S = Sunni; H = Shi'a; D = Druze)
*Less than 20 cases in base

Figure 8. The effect of wife's education on the proportion of wives who ever used contraception by religious affiliation net of marriage duration, marriage age, parity, income, husband's occupation, and size of place of residence: Lebanon, 1971.

To determine whether or not differences in past and current contraceptive use are simply the product of background differences among the religious groups, we again rely on regression techniques. For both past and current contraceptive use, the addition of an interaction term contributes significantly to the proportion of the variance explained; therefore, wife's education and religion are regarded as a single predictor in the MCA analyses.

Of all the independent variables, wife's education × religion, *WE* × *R*, has by far the greatest effect on past and current contraceptive use (Tables A.10 and A.11). *WE* × *R*'s squared multiple partial coefficients for past and current contraceptive use are 10.7 and 7.3 percent, respectively. The influences of marriage duration and parity, the second most important set of variables, are substantially less (4.1 and 2.3 percent, respectively). The effects of marriage age, total family income, husband's occupation, and size of place of residence are relatively small. The pattern of their influences, however, is generally as expected. For example, contraceptive use varies directly with size of place of residence: (1) 72 percent for places with 10,000 or more inhabitants; (2)

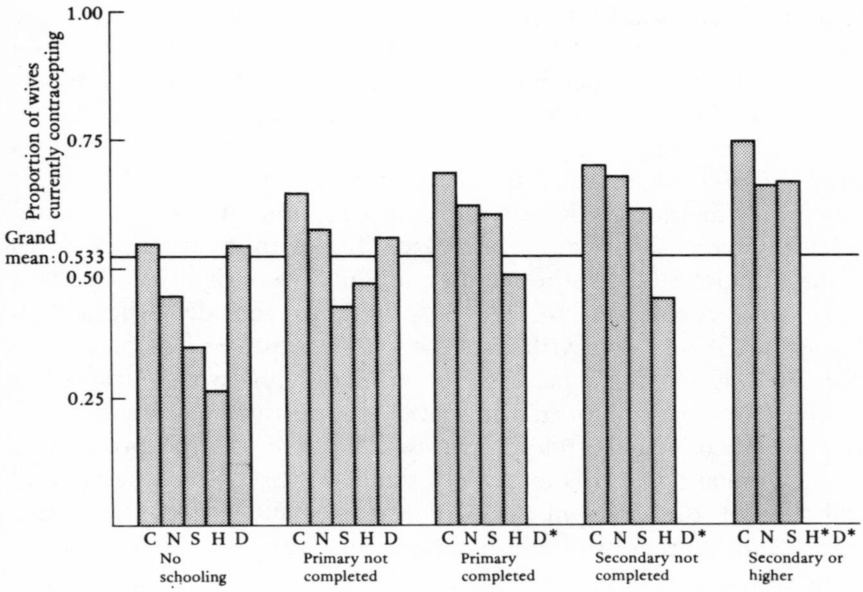

Note: Religion by wife's education (C = Catholic; N = Non-Catholic Christian; S = Sunni; H = Shi'a; D = Druze)
*Less than 20 cases in base

Figure 9. The effect of wife's education on the proportion of wives currently contracepting by religious affiliation net of marriage duration, marriage age, parity, income, husband's occupation, and size of place of residence: Lebanon, 1971.

64 percent for places with 1,000 to 9,999 inhabitants; and (3) 55 percent for places with less than 1,000 inhabitants.

Our MCA results also indicate that religious differences in contraceptive use are inversely related to wife's education. The largest differences generally occur among wives with no schooling, and the smallest among wives with secondary school or higher completed (Figures 8 and 9). For example, whereas the Catholic–Sunni difference in past contraceptive use is 23.3 percent for wives with no schooling, it is only 3.8 percent for wives with secondary or higher education. Moreover, in comparison to the non-Catholic Christians, the proportions for the Sunnis are actually somewhat greater at the highest levels of wife's education.

These results also demonstrate that the observed religious differences in contraceptive use among the Lebanese couples are associated, to a large extent, with differences in educational status among the sects. If the sects were to have the same educational distributions but to retain their individual rates (the gross effects in Tables A.10 and A.11), the overall proportions for the sects would become considerably more alike. For example, if the Sunnis were to have the educational distribution of the non-Catholic Christians and to retain their own rates, the overall proportion of past contraceptive use for the Sunnis would increase from 62 to 72 percent, which compares extremely well to the overall proportion of 73 percent for the non-Catholic Christians.

In an earlier section of this chapter, we found that the religious groups, net of background differences, differed in their knowledge of contraceptive methods. Whereas the Catholics, non-Catholic Christians, and Druzes were significantly more familier with coitus interruptus than the Sunnis or Shi'as. the Sunnis and Shi'as were significantly more familiar with tubal ligation. We now wish to consider whether an analogous situation exists with respect to contraceptive practice.

Our analysis of this issue focuses primarily on two contraceptive methods. Our measure of traditional contraceptive use is again the proportion practicing coitus interruptus. However, as the proportion who had a tubal ligation is extremely small (about 1 percent), we rely on the use of the oral pill as an indicator of modern contraceptive practice. Both of these variables concern current use of the methods at the time of the interview.

As was noted earlier, the Catholics, non-Catholic Christians, and Druzes were currently using coitus interruptus to a significantly greater extent than were the Sunnis or Shi'as: (1) Catholics, 40 percent; (2) Druzes, 33 percent; (3) non-Catholic Christians, 32 percent; (4) Sunnis, 20 percent; and (5) Shi'as, 10 percent. Though these differences remain essentially unchanged within most age and age-parity categories, they are strongly influenced by wife's education (Table 10).

The largest religious differences in the use of coitus interruptus are found among wives who have not completed primary school. At this level, the proportions for the Catholics, non-Catholic Christians, and Druzes are two to three times larger than the proportions for the Shi'as and Sunnis. In contrast, the differences are considerably less among wives who completed secondary school or higher. Moreover, the division among the religious groups is not clear-cut. At the higher educational levels, the proportion who were using coitus interruptus for Sunnis is similar to or greater than that for the non-Catholic Christians. For example, although among wives 15 to 29 years old who had not completed primary school, the proportions for non-Catholic Christians and Sunnis are 33 and 15 percent, respectively, the proportions for the same age group at the highest educational level are 7 and 15 percent, respectively.

Table 10. *Proportion of wives currently using coitus interruptus by religion, wife's age, and wife's education: Lebanon, 1971*

Wife's education by wife's age	Religion: Catholic	Non-Catholic Christian	Sunni	Shi'a	Druze	Total
15–29						
Primary not completed	39	33	15	8	23	21
Secondary not completed	35	17	22	13	*	25
Secondary or higher completed	24	7	15	*	*	17
30–49						
Primary not completed	41	39	20	10	42	28
Secondary not completed	47	36	33	*	*	40
Secondary or higher completed	27	20	18	*	*	23
All wives	40	32	20	10	33	27
N	921	590	563	566	119	2,759

*Less than 20 cases in base

Due to their higher socioeconomic levels, we had also expected that the Catholic and non-Catholic Christian couples would exhibit higher usage of the oral pill than the Sunnis and Shi'as. The results of the *NFFP* survey indicate just the opposite. Sunnis and Shi'as had the greatest proportions currently using the oral pill: (1) Sunnis, 20 percent; (2) Shi'as, 17 percent; (3) Druzes, 15 percent; (4) non-Catholic Christians, 12 percent; and (5) Catholics, 10 percent.

Controlling for wife's education and age does not seriously modify the higher proportions of oral pill usage among Sunnis and Shi'as (Table 11). Only among wives 15 to 29 years old who had not completed primary school are the proportions for the non-Catholic Christians and Druzes greater than the Sunni proportion (11, 13, and 10 percent, respectively). In all other comparisons, the proportions for Sunnis and Shi'as are larger than those for the other groups.

Table 11. *Proportion of wives currently using oral pill by religion, wife's age, and wife's education: Lebanon, 1971*

Wife's education by wife's age	Religion: Catholic	Non-Catholic Christian	Sunni	Shi'a	Druze	Total
15–29						
Primary not completed	9	11	10	16	13	11
Secondary not completed	12	17	33	29	*	20
Secondary or higher completed	24	21	26	*	*	22
30–49						
Primary not completed	8	7	20	16	10	12
Secondary not completed	13	18	25	*	*	18
Secondary or higher completed	15	13	36	*	*	16
All wives	10	12	20	17	15	14
N	921	590	563	566	119	2,759

*Less than 20 cases in base

In brief, for the two Christian groups wife's education is fairly strongly and consistently negatively correlated to the use of coitus interruptus and positively correlated to the use of the oral pill. Among the Muslim groups, in contrast, there is no consistent pattern between wife's education and the use of coitus interruptus, but there is, as with Christians, a positive relationship between wife's education and the use of the oral pill. These constituent patterns lie behind the trends in total contraceptive use described earlier (Figures 8 and 9). Coitus interruptus, a method that has been in use for centuries, is practiced most by the Christian groups at every educational level, but is especially preeminent among the poorly educated. The more highly educated couples among both the Christian and Muslim sects are taking up the oral pill, although, interestingly enough, there is a large residual group of better-educated Christians who continue to practice coitus interruptus.

7. Summary and conclusions

Summary

This investigation began with a discussion of the relevance of religion to fertility and then turned to a review of the three major theoretical explanations for religious differences in fertility: the characteristics hypothesis, the particularized theology proposition, and the minority group status hypothesis. In brief, the advocates of the characteristics hypothesis contend that religious differences in fertility are simply the result of differences in the demographic, social, and economic attributes of the members of the religious groups. If the attributes of the groups were similar, this hypothesis maintains, the religious fertility differentials would be negligible. Supporters of the particularized theology proposition, in contrast, maintain that religious differentials in fertility are due to differences in church doctrines or ideology on fertility control and family size. Accordingly, religious groups whose ideologies prohibit the use of contraception and abortion and emphasize the value of many children should demonstrate higher fertility than groups whose ideologies permit contraception and do not stress the importance of many children. Finally, the proponents of the minority group status hypothesis posit that under certain circumstances, the insecurities of minority group status depress fertility below majority levels.

The lack of congruence between the existing theoretical explanations and the results of empirical studies led us to propose a hypothesis that not only offers a broader conceptual framework within which to understand religious differentials in fertility, but also appears to be more generally consistent with the results of previous research. Our proposition, which we call the interaction hypothesis, contends that religious fertility differentials are largely a function of two broad factors: (1) the doctrines and the current, local orientations of the religions involved; and (2) the socioeconomic levels of the religious groups considered. In brief, the interaction hypothesis maintains that religious values and orientations that are pronatalist have their principal effect during the demographic transition because their influence produces a lag in the adjustment of their members' fertility to the conditions for which low fertility is an appropriate modification. Before the demographic transition high fertility is appropriate for everyone, so religion does not differentiate. After the transition, the religious influence is eventually negated by the conditions of modern society.

As mentioned previously, the data under investigation are from the 1971 National Fertility and Family Planning Survey (*NFFP*) conducted by the Lebanon Family Planning Association. This probability sample of Lebanese couples, with wives 15 to 49 years old ($N = 2{,}795$), is well suited for an inquiry into religious differentials in fertility not only because of the considerable religious heterogeneity in Lebanon, but also because of the absence of significant racial and ethnic differences among the Lebanese.

As the Lebanese data were taken from a society at a single point in time, we did not expect to encounter the entire pattern of religious fertility differentials as specified by the interaction hypothesis. Taking into consideration Lebanon's intermediate level of development, and controlling for demographic differences such as marriage duration, wife's age, and residence status, religious differentials in fertility among the Lebanese were expected to be greatest among the lower socioeconomic classes and smallest among the higher socioeconomic classes, with the religious groups with the more pronatalist orientations having the higher fertility.

With respect to the positions of the religious groups on procreation and fertility control, we differentiated between the official religious doctrines of a sect or group and its particular local orientation, by which we mean the current attitudes and views toward fertility and fertility control prevailing among a religious community. Reliance on the official church doctrines tends to mislead one in ascertaining the extent of pronatalism among the groups, and therefore we chose the local orientations of the groups as indicators of their religious positions. Based upon their political histories, migratory patterns, differing associations and affiliations, and other factors that help to shape the local religious community's attitudes and views on fertility and birth control, the two Christian groups were believed to be less pronatalist in their positions on procreation and fertility control than the Muslims, and among the Muslims, the Druzes were thought to be less pronatalist than the Sunnis or Shi'as.

The first step in our empirical investigation of religious fertility differentials was to establish the extent of fertility differences within and between the two major faiths in Lebanon. Contrary to Yaukey's (1961) findings for Lebanon, we found significant fertility differences among the Muslims (Sunnis, Shi'as, and Druzes) and among Christians (Catholics and non-Catholic Christians). Consequently, throughout our research, data on each of the five religious groups were analyzed separately. The relative ranking of the religious groups from high to low fertility (for both period and cohort fertility) was: Shi'as, Sunnis, Druzes and Catholics, and non-Catholic Christians.

Owing to the substantial background differences among the religious groups and the small numbers of cases in many of the categories, additive models employing regression techniques were utilized in order to determine the net effects of religion on fertility. The regression analyses found the interaction term of wife's education × religion ($WE \times R$) to be significant for number of children ever born (NOCEB) and number of living children (NLC), but not for the proportion of women who had a live birth in 1970 (LB70). For NOCEB and NLC, this meant that religious fertility differentials were not constant across educational categories. At low levels of wife's education, differentials were great, with Sunnis and Shi'as having considerably higher fertility than the Druzes, Catholics, and non-Catholic Christians. At high levels of wife's education, religious differentials were insignificant. In contrast, the analyses of LB70 indicated constant fertility differences by wife's education among the five groups, with the ranking of the groups much the same as without controls. These findings, however, were considered less credible due to the statistical shortcomings inherent in the use of a highly skewed dichotomous dependent variable.

After having concluded that the religious fertility differentials were a function of the interaction of wife's education and the local orientations of the religious groups, the next step in the investigation was to look more closely at the specific ways in which differences in religious affiliation are translated into fertility differentials. According to the determinants of fertility framework of Davis and Blake (1956) and Freedman (1967) (Figure 1), the effects of religious affiliation on fertility operate via the norms about family size and the norms about the intermediate variables as well as through the intermediate variables themselves. Assuming appropriate controls for demographic, social, and economic characteristics, the net fertility differentials among the religious groups are thought to arise largely from two sources: (1) religious differences in the number of children wanted; and (2) religious differences in the willingness and ability to limit fertility.

Regression analyses and cross-tabulation methods yielded identical results for the relationship between religion and family size preferences. In contrast to the measures of completed fertility, the interaction term for religious affiliation and wife's education was not significant for family size preferences. In other words, the effects of religious affiliation on family size preferences did not depend on the level of wife's education. Shi'as expressed larger family size ideals and desired substantially more additional children than any of the other religious groups. Although there were differences in family size preferences among the Sunnis, Druzes, Catholics, and non-Catholic Christians, these differences were relatively minor in relation to comparisons involving Shi'as.

With the exception of wives with no schooling, we found that religious differences in attitudes toward fertility control were minor. Regardless of religious affiliation, the large majority of wives with some schooling approved of the use of contraceptive methods and desired further information about family planning. Among wives with no schooling, however, Sunnis and Shi'as were significantly less approving of contraception than were Catholics, non-Catholic Christians, and Druzes.

Religious differences in knowledge of fertility control were not as straightforward among the religious groups as were attitudinal differences in fertility control. Among illiterate and poorly educated women, the two Christian groups were more knowledgeable about traditional methods; however, this was not so among well-educated women. For example, religious differences in knowledge of coitus interruptus among wives who completed high school or higher levels were minor. Religious differences in knowledge of tubal ligation, in contrast, did not follow the pattern noted for coitus interruptus. Shi'as and Sunnis were more familiar with tubal ligation than were Catholics, non-Catholic Christians, and Druzes, and these differences broadened with increases in wife's education.

Religious differences in fertility control practice (ever used and current use of contraception) were consistent with the pattern of religious fertility differentials. At the lower levels of wife's education religious differences in contraceptive practice were large, with Sunnis and Shi'as reporting the lowest rates of contraceptive usage. At high levels of wife's education, religious differences in contraceptive practice were minor. However, there were significant religious differences in the contraceptive methods employed. Catholics, non-Catholic Christians, and Druzes used traditional methods (primarily coitus interruptus) to a greater extent than did Sunnis and Shi'as, who relied more heavily on the oral pill. These results and those regarding religious differences in knowledge of contraceptives suggested a traditional–modern contraceptive division between Catholics, non-Catholic Christians, and Druzes on the one hand, and Sunnis and Shi'as on the other.

Conclusions

Among the major findings of this research, one of the most evident is that simple Muslim–Christian comparisons are not particularly meaningful. Within each of the two major faiths, important differences in fertility, family size preferences, and knowledge, attitudes, and practices of fertility control were observed among the sects. In many instances the averages of the proportions for the Christian groups fell in between or were divided by the corresponding figures for the Muslim sects. In more than a few cases, intrafaith comparisons yielded differentials that were as large or larger than those obtained from interfaith comparisons. In light of this evidence, to continue to speak of and to make decisions on the basis of simple Muslim–Christian differences is not only unreasonable, but also misleading.

Except for the Shi'as, differences in family size preferences appeared to play almost no role in accounting for net fertility differences, as the groups wanted roughly the same number of children. Family size preference as a source of fertility differentials, however, cannot be totally ruled out because there is no way in which to assess the differential intensity of commitment to these expressed preferences.

Only among illiterate and poorly educated wives were net fertility differentials found to be significant between the Sunnis vis-à-vis the Catholics, non-Catholic Christians, and Druzes. The evidence suggests that these differentials were not due to differences in family size preferences, but were primarily the result of differences in knowledge and practice of birth control. Given the greater availability of contraceptive information and methods, the fertility of the Sunnis is likely to decrease rapidly to a level commensurate with their family size preferences.

In contrast to the Sunnis, the differentials in fertility between the Shi'as and the other religious groups were congruent with differences in both family size preferences and willingness and ability to limit fertility. Despite controls for demographic, social, and economic variables, the Shi'as expressed the largest family size ideals and wanted the greatest number of additional children. Among illiterate and poorly educated wives, the Shi'as were the least knowledgeable about contraceptives, were the least approving of fertility control, and had the lowest levels of contraceptive use. At these low levels of education, the fertility differentials between the Shi'as and the other groups were by far the largest. The higher the educational status of the Shi'a subgroups the greater were the knowledge, attitudes, and practices of fertility control, and the smaller were the religious differentials in fertility.

The net fertility differentials among the Catholics, non-Catholic Christians, and Druzes were relatively small. This is consistent with the similarities both of their family size preferences and of their willingness and ability to limit their fertility. The net fertility differentials that did exist among these groups are likely to be associated with aspects of family size preferences and family limitation that were not measured in the *NFFP* survey – for example, duration of contraceptive use and commitment to preferences.

An unexpected finding of our investigation, but one that was also encountered in the WHO (1976) study, was the significant differences in the contraceptive methods known and utilized among the religious groups. Quite paradoxically, the groups with the more modern social and economic characteristics (the Catholics and non-Catholic Christians) relied more heavily on traditional methods such as coitus interruptus, and the groups with the more traditional characteristics (the Sunnis and Shi'as) used modern methods such as the oral pill to a greater extent. For example, the Sunnis and Shi'as were substantially more familiar with tubal ligation than were the other groups. Furthermore, controlling for wife's education and other background characteristics increased these differences somewhat, rather than reducing them as might have been expected.

One plausible explanation for this peculiar division is that due to their greater contact with the French and their migratory patterns to and from the West, the Christian groups began their contraceptive practices earlier than the Sunnis and Shi'as. In this earlier period, coitus interruptus and other traditional methods were the only means of contraception available; consequently, the Christian groups relied and continue to rely heavily on these techniques. As the Sunnis and Shi'as did not have a history of reliance on these methods, these Muslim groups were perhaps more likely to adopt the more advanced contraceptive methods than were the Christian groups, whose contraceptive practices were already relatively firmly established.

One especially valuable lesson to be gained from our inquiry which cannot be stressed too strongly is the error of generalizing from the official doctrines and theology of a religion to the fertility behavior of its members. Researchers studying the effects of Islam on fertility, as well as policymakers who base their decision making on this research, have been much more prone to commit this error than those examining the effects of Christianity or Judaism on fertility. Although consideration of a religious text and its interpretations may be a useful endeavor in an analysis of the evolution of religious beliefs, habits, and attitudes, reliance on them as an explanation of current fertility behavior is likely to lead one astray. Rather than depending on interpretations of Koranic verses, Hadiths, official statements, and other such ideological materials, social scientists, religious leaders, and those persons involved in the formulation of population policy should rely upon the current local orientations of the particular religious groups toward fertility and birth control for a proper understanding of the dynamics of their fertility behavior.

Another important finding of this research that is of particular significance for countries in the Middle East is that in the multireligious Arab country of Lebanon, the indexes of modernization were related to fertility, family size preferences, and knowledge, attitudes, and practices of fertility control after allowing for the effects of religion. Regardless of which religious group was considered, it was generally the case that total family income, husband's occupational status, wife's education, and size of place of residence were positively related to fertility control. These results should be viewed as encouraging by those who are concerned with the rapid rates of population growth in the Middle Eastern countries.

These findings also have important implications for population policymakers in countries where religious composition is a sensitive issue. First, they should realize that religion is an important characteristic in differentiating fertility behavior, but only at certain socioeconomic levels. Second, large religious differentials in fertility may be reduced substantially, and relatively rapidly, with improvements in the social and economic statuses of the less advantaged religious groups. Without such improvements, however, large fertility differentials among religious groups may lead to considerable alterations in a population's religious composition, which in turn may have dramatic effects on a country's existing political system and overall stability.

There are also important theoretical implications emanating from our investigation. It appears evident that in themselves the particularized theology proposition, the characteristics hypothesis, and the minority group status hypothesis are not sufficiently satisfactory explanations for the observed Lebanese religious differentials in fertility. Contrary to the hypothesis of the particularized position, the pattern of the fertility differences among the religious groups was not at all consistent with the official positions and ideologies of the religions. For example, the Catholics, the group with the most pronatalist official position, demonstrated the second lowest fertility of the five religious groups.

Equally apparent is the inadequacy of the characteristics proposition. The fertility differentials among the religious groups are not simply reflections of the social, demographic, or economic attributes of the members of the religious groups. There are significant and important differences in these groups' characteristics, but these differences by themselves cannot fully account for the fertility differentials.

The minority group status hypothesis also appears unacceptable as an explanation for the religious fertility differentials. In a country such as Lebanon it is not at all apparent which of the religious groups should be viewed as the minority. It is not evident whether minority status should be decided on the basis of the relative size of the sect or major faith, by socioeconomic status, or by access to political power. Except for the Armenians, the concept of acculturation that is heavily relied upon in this hypothesis is also not appropriate in the case of Lebanon. Members of the religious groups are not in the process of acquiring "Lebanese" cultural traits; the members are indigenous to the area and culture. Furthermore, the effect of a minority group's status (according to size) on fertility at the district level was not useful in explaining religious fertility differentials. Residing in a district where one's religious group is a clear numerical minority was found to have no significant or consistent impact on fertility.

In contrast to the previous propositions, the interaction hypothesis is largely supported by the results of our analyses. As was hypothesized, fertility differentials among the religious groups decreased as the socioeconomic status of the couples increased. This pattern was found for number of children ever born, and for number of living children, but not for the proportion of women who had a live birth in 1970. Employing wife's education as our measure of socioeconomic status and controlling for a number of demographic, social, and economic factors, we observed that the religious differentials in cumulative fertility depended on the level of wife's education. At low levels of wife's education fertility differentials were large, but at high levels of wife's education religious fertility differentials were negligible.

We also expected that the Lebanese groups with the more pronatalist current local orientations would have higher fertility, especially at lower levels of socioeconomic status. More specifically, we predicted that Sunnis and Shi'as would demonstrate the highest fertility, Catholics and non-Catholic Christians the lowest fertility, and Druzes the intermediate fertility. In fact, this was precisely the ordering observed at lower levels of wife's education.

It is interesting to note briefly in passing (to do any more would be difficult given the quality of the available data) that, if we also consider some of the results of Yaukey's (1961) 1958 study, a great portion of the pattern of religious fertility differentials described by the interaction hypothesis may be observed. Namely, Yaukey found that rural Christians demonstrated essentially the same fertility as rural Muslims but that Muslims showed higher fertility in the urban areas. When Yaukey's findings are combined with ours they suggest a picture that is at least not inconsistent with the pattern specified by the interaction hypotheses – that is, the absence of religious fertility differentials at the lowest and highest socioeconomic levels and their presence at intermediate socioeconomic levels. It does appear that the interaction hypothesis potentially provides a reasonable explanation for the observed fertility differentials among the religious groups in Lebanon.

One of the most prominent issues raised by our investigation is whether the interaction hypothesis can assist in the explanation of religious differentials in fertility in countries other than Lebanon. Although to answer this question properly data are needed in a form such that they adequately take into account demographic, social, and economic differences in the characteristics of the religious groups, sufficient research does exist to suggest strongly that the interaction hypothesis is generalizable.

There are several sets of data in the United States, for instance, that support the interaction hypothesis. As mentioned previously, for example, Mayer and Marx (1957) found that over the period from 1920 to 1950 the fertility of Polish Catholics in Hamtramck, Michigan, converged rapidly toward the fertility of the general U.S. population. In Rhode Island for the period of 1967 to 1971, Bouvier and Rao (1975) found a convergence in the fertility behavior and attitudes of Catholics and Protestants. Also, as we noted earlier, Westoff and Jones (1978) observed when looking over the five national studies of fertility and family planning that the fact of being a Catholic has become virtually insignificant as a determinant of fertility, attitudes toward fertility control, and the practice of contraception. Ryder (1973) also reported that differences for wanted fertility, for unwanted fertility, and for the specific modes of fertility regulation have diminished appreciably among religious groups in the United States during the past decade.

Although the fertility measures are crude and there are no controls for the substantial social and economic differences in the characteristics of the religious groups, the religious fertility differentials that existed in Prussia from 1842 to 1934 also appear to be generally consistent with the interaction hypothesis. In Figure 10 we illustrate the crude birthrates for Prussian Catholics, Protestants, and Jews during the period from 1842 to 1934 (Knodel 1974, p. 137). From 1842 to 1844, the fertility levels of the three groups were relatively similar (between 37 and 41 per 1,000). From 1842 to 1865 the fertility of the Catholics and Protestants remained unchanged, although Jewish fertility began to decline. The fertility differences among the religious groups then expanded in the period from 1858 to 1910. After 1910, with the exception of the sudden drop in the Jewish birthrate between 1924 and 1934, there is some indication of a convergence in the rates among the religious groups. More recent comparisons of Catholic and Protestant marriage cohorts in the Federal Republic of Germany, based on the 1950 census, indicate a progressive contraction of the differential for successive marriage cohorts. For the most recent cohort examined (1937–1940), the difference disappeared in localities of 100,000 or more inhabitants, although in smaller localities Catholics showed slightly higher fertility (Schwarz 1965).

Our final example of where the pattern of religious differentials in fertility is consistent with the interaction hypothesis is the Netherlands. As mentioned earlier, Van Praag and Lohle-Tart (1974) found that fertility differentials that had existed between Catholics and Protestants

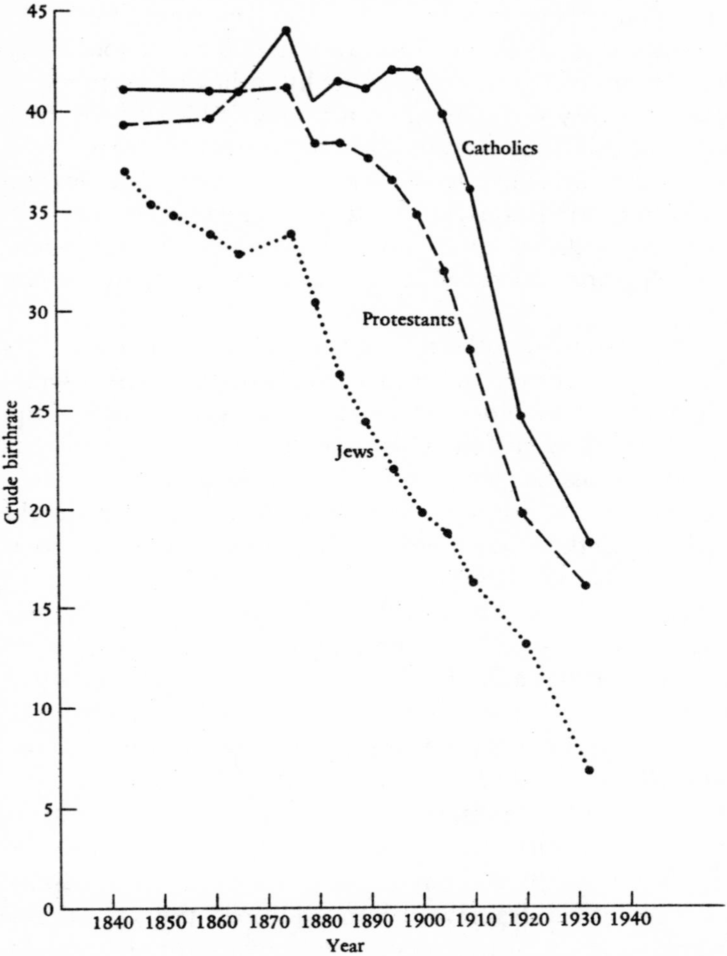

Figure 10. Crude birthrates for Catholics, Protestants, and Jews: Prussia, 1842–1934.

in the Netherlands were insignificant by the late sixties. Because of a much faster fertility decline in the Catholic provinces, a 16 percent differential in marital fertility around 1960 was more than wiped out by 1967 (p. 304). Furthermore, the recent evidence from the 1975 Netherlands Survey on Fertility and Parenthood Motivation continues to show the absence of religious fertility differentials (Moors 1978).

As is true of most theories or hypotheses, the interaction hypothesis, while attempting to answer certain questions, has raised other issues.

Among these there are three that are relatively important. First, the interaction hypothesis as it is presently formulated lacks specificity with respect to its time reference. Because the hypothesis does not spell out when religious fertility differentials will be negligible, it is possible to maintain, for example, that current differentials will be insignificant sometime in the future. Certainly what is needed is greater specification of the socioeconomic conditions under which religious fertility differentials will be observed. No doubt this will depend to a great extent on the particular religions concerned as well as on the particular sociocultural setting.

Second, the interaction hypothesis is oversimplified when it comes to actually describing what may occur in a given situation. The interaction hypothesis does not include factors that may greatly affect the pattern of religious fertility differentials in a particular country – that is, group cohesion, cross-national linkages, political upheavals and conflicts, migration, natural disasters, and so forth. However, it should be added that the hypothesis does not preclude the inclusion of such factors in explaining specific cases.

Third, in its current form the hypothesis is unable to specify the pathways by which fertility will decline among the religious groups. Experience in Asia, Europe, and the Far East indicates that there are numerous different blends of the "intermediate variables" that a population may demonstrate in moving from high to low fertility (Davis 1963; Coale 1969; World Bank 1974; Bongaarts 1978).

Nevertheless, despite these limitations, the interaction hypothesis is helpful in explaining religious fertility differentials. For instance, the hypothesis brings together a large body of previously conflicting results within a broad theoretical framework. In addition, the hypothesis stresses the local orientations of the religious groups toward procreation and fertility control rather than the official religious doctrines or laws. As mentioned previously, this distinction is important, as it is often the case that a sect may have an official position that differs greatly from the attitudes and practices existing among its followers and clergy. Furthermore, the hypothesis is not limited to viewing religious fertility differentials at a single point in time; it places the differentials within a historical perspective. Such a context is superior to cross-sectional theoretical explanations, for as we found earlier, religious differentials in fertility do not remain constant over time.

In conclusion, although this investigation has generally omitted discussion of the tragic events that have recently occurred in Lebanon, this should in no way be construed to mean that the findings are unrelated to the Lebanese conflict.[1] On the contrary, there are very few countries in the world in which demography is so directly, fundamentally, and intimately linked to the official distribution of political power.[2] We indicated earlier that the Lebanese constitution stipulates that the Chamber of Deputies is to be elected by the population in such a manner that it is proportionately representative of the various confessional communities. In addition, top governmental positions and appointments throughout the bureaucracy are tied by rigid tradition to a sect's relative numerical size (e.g., the office of the president to the largest sect, the prime ministership to the second largest, and so on).

Under such circumstances, it is not surprising that the stability of the Lebanese sociopolitical system has been significantly affected by the sizable fertility differentials among the religious groups. Differential rates of fertility have corresponded closely to religious differences in growth rates, which in turn have altered the relative demographic standings of the religious groups and consequently have challenged the existing distribution of political power and advantage among the groups. To be more specific, assuming a somewhat higher crude death rate for Shi'as and Sunnis than for the others, namely, 9 per 1,000 for Shi'as and Sunnis and 7 per 1,000 for Catholics, Druzes, and non-Catholic Christians; and translating the observed total fertility rates to crude birthrates, that is, birthrates of 47 per 1,000 for Shi'as, 37 for Sunnis, 27 for Catholics, 25 for Druzes, and 24 for non-Catholic Christians;[3] we obtain the following rates of natural increase for the five religious groups: Shi'as, 3.8 percent; Sunnis, 2.8 percent; Catholics, 2.0 percent; Druzes, 1.8 percent; and non-Catholic Christians, 1.7 percent.

Moreover, if the migration patterns of the sects are taken into account, the differences in the growth rates are likely to be greater. Although accurate emigration figures are not available, several studies (Safa 1960; Khuri 1967, 1975) have shown that members of Christian denominations are more likely to emigrate than members of the Muslim sects, which is reasonable given the sizable socioeconomic differences among the groups.

What do the more rapid rates of growth of the Sunnis and, in particular, the Shi'as imply for the Lebanese political system? To begin with, in theory at least, these differential growth rates point to a redistribution of seats in the Chamber of Deputies in favor of the Muslims, who are undoubtedly much more numerous than the Christians. Furthermore, among the Muslims the majority of deputy seats would not go to the

Sunnis, but to the Shi'as. In other words, the Chamber would be under the control of the generally less wealthy Muslims, and the sect with the greatest number of seats in the Chamber would be the Shi'as, who are the poorest, least educated, and, historically, the most disfranchised of the Lebanese religious groups.

Potentially even more significant than the adjustments in the Chamber are the implications that these differential growth rates have regarding the distribution of the top governmental offices. If the practice of allocating high government offices according to the size of a sect is adhered to, the Maronites, for example, would not even be entitled to the office of the prime minister, which would be retained by the Sunnis, the second largest sect; the highest office available to the Maronites would probably be the speaker of the Chamber of Deputies. The office of the presidency would be the domain of the Shi'as, the largest single sect. In brief, if the political structure properly reflected the religious composition of the population, as it constitutionally and traditionally has been set up to do, then the Muslims, and especially the Shi'as, would inherit enormous political power and advantage. Conversely, the Christians, and in particular the Maronites, would have to give up much of their official political dominance.

Of course, the Lebanese civil war has so drastically altered the Lebanese political scene that it is difficult to imagine the form that the political system will have in the future. The principal value in considering theoretically what the Lebanese system would or might be is to gain a better understanding of: (1) the interplay between demographic phenomena on the one hand, and political behavior on the other, and (2) the effects of this interplay on the socioeconomic and political system as a whole. In the specific case of Lebanon, it seems evident that significant changes in the religious composition of the population in the absence of commensurate changes in the distribution of political and governmental power contributed to a great extent, both directly as well as indirectly, to the civil war. It also seems clear that the changes that have occurred in the country's religious composition currently provide a partial explanation of why a number of the more powerful Maronite groups are unwilling to return to a demographically modified, prewar political system and are strongly advocating partition of a loosely tied confederation. For if these groups were to agree to a modified, prewar system, then they would in fact be saying that they are willing to give up much of their official political power and dominance as well as related social and economic advantages. At present, they are unwilling to do so.

More generally, the experience of Lebanon indicates that if a multireligious (or multiethnic) society wishes to operate within a confessional system of government based on proportionate representation, then significant changes in the composition of the population must be recognized and satisfactorily reflected within governmental and political structures. To do otherwise is almost certain to lead to alienation, frustration, and violence, as it has in Lebanon.

Appendix A. Supplementary tables

Table A.1. *Gross and net effects of demographic, social, and economic variables on number of children ever born: Lebanon, 1971*

Independent variables	N	Gross effect	R^2	Net effect	R^2
Marriage duration (years)			.440		.373
0–4	445	−3.283		−2.984	
5–9	520	−1.420		−1.360	
10–14	639	.055		.077	
15–19	448	1.361		1.263	
20+	700	2.221		2.029	
Age at marriage (years)			.062		.001
12–16	575	.983		.080	
17–19	786	.398		.178	
20–21	480	−.339		−.075	
22–24	461	−.546		−.014	
25+	425	−1.138		−.310	
Not ascertained	25	.794		−.481	
Wife's education × *religion*			.217		.132
No schooling:					
Catholic	265	1.019		.062	
Non-Catholic Christian	122	.667		−.198	
Sunni	272	1.262		.938	
Shi'a	390	2.070		1.453	
Druze	28	−.223		−.255	
Primary not completed:					
Catholic	277	−.355		−.566	
Non-Catholic Christian	189	−.493		−.810	
Sunni	133	.559		.484	
Shi'a	109	.248		.755	
Druze	51	−.111		−.114	

Table A.1. *(cont.)*

Independent variables	N	Gross effect	R^2	Net effect	R^2
Primary completed:					
Catholic	170	-1.307		-.818	
Non-Catholic Christian	114	-1.436		-1.002	
Sunni	66	.028		.292	
Shi'a	30	-.800		.397	
Druze	13	*		*	
Secondary not completed:					
Catholic	124	-1.649		-.615	
Non-Catholic Christian	83	-1.788		-1.500	
Sunni	44	-1.911		-.617	
Shi'a	20	-1.566		.039	
Druze	11	*		*	
Secondary or higher completed:					
Catholic	80	-2.316		-.815	
Non-Catholic Christian	82	-1.964		-.703	
Sunni	48	-2.241		-.821	
Shi'a	15	*		*	
Druze	16	*		*	
Total family income (Lebanese pounds)			.046		.002
0–2,999	939	.639		-.001	
3,000–5,999	754	.016		.077	
6,000–9,999	336	-.447		-.047	
10,000–14,999	184	-1.400		-.276	
15,000+	212	-1.111		-.284	
Not ascertained	327	.120		.213	
Husband's occupation			.081		.009
Professional/technical	120	-1.916		-.469	
Business/management	460	-.434		-.192	
Clerical/sales	336	-1.027		-.116	
Police/army/guard	172	-.390		.076	
Crafts/operatives	557	-.097		.064	
Farming	238	1.134		.165	
Labor	592	.740		.081	
Peddlery	47	1.889		.834	
Other	160	-.041		.091	
Not ascertained	70	1.505		-.079	

Table A.1. *(cont.)*

Independent variables	N	Gross effect	R^2	Net effect	R^2
Size of place of residence			.012		.006
10,000+	1,603	-.244		-.149	
1,000 to 9,999	630	.151		.225	
Less than 1,000	519	.570		.188	
R^2 for total equation	2,752		.563		

Notes: The grand mean for NOCEB is 4.367. Gross effect coefficients are deviations of the category raw means from the grand mean; and the net effect coefficients, or regression coefficients, are the deviations of the category means from the grand mean net of the effects of the other explanatory variables. The gross effect R^2 is eta squared based on MCA, and the net effect R^2 is the squared multiple partial coefficient based on dummy variable regression.

*Less than 20 cases in base.

Table A.2. *Gross and net effects of demographic, social, and economic variables on number of living children: Lebanon, 1971*

Independent variables	N	Gross effect	R^2	Net effect	R^2
Marriage duration (years)			.431		.342
0–4	445	-3.000		-2.750	
5–9	520	-1.211		-1.175	
10–14	639	.145		.162	
15–19	448	1.279		1.198	
20+	700	1.855		1.707	
Age at marriage (years)			.058		.002
12–16	575	.828		.060	
17–19	786	.361		.172	
20–21	480	-.263		-.035	
22–24	461	-.463		-.012	
25+	425	-1.017		-.316	
Not ascertained	25	.482		-.550	
Wife's education X *religion*			.192		.109
No schooling:					
Catholic	265	.920		.099	
Non-Catholic Christian	122	.568		-.172	
Sunni	272	1.010		.749	
Shi'a	390	1.672		1.140	
Druze	28	-.145		-.170	

Table A.2. *(cont.)*

Independent variables	N	Gross effect	R^2	Net effect	R^2
Primary not completed:					
Catholic	277	-.226		-.428	
Non-Catholic Christian	189	-.440		-.711	
Sunni	133	.511		.442	
Shi'a	109	.301		.728	
Druze	51	-.019		.010	
Primary completed:					
Catholic	170	-1.110		-.702	
Non-Catholic Christian	114	-1.222		-.849	
Sunni	66	.113		.332	
Shi'a	30	-.605		.447	
Druze	13	*		*	
Secondary not completed:					
Catholic	124	-1.385		-.482	
Non-Catholic Christian	83	-1.508		-1.275	
Sunni	44	-1.675		-.527	
Shi'a	20	-1.288		.098	
Druze	11	*		*	
Secondary or higher completed:					
Catholic	80	-2.013		-.704	
Non-Catholic Christian	82	-1.733		-.642	
Sunni	48	-1.955		-.746	
Shi'a	15	*		*	
Druze	16	*		*	
Total family income (Lebanese pounds)			.038		.001
0–2,999	939	.489		-.041	
3,000–5,999	754	.035		.075	
6,000–9,999	336	-.312		.022	
10,000–14,999	184	-1.190		-.215	
15,000+	212	-.897		-.181	
Not ascertained	327	.087		.159	
Husband's occupation			.070		.009
Professional/technical	120	-1.638		-.399	
Business/management	460	-.343		-.156	
Clerical/sales	336	-.877		-.110	
Police/army/guard	172	-.288		.068	
Crafts/operatives	557	-.056		.069	
Farming	238	.907		.095	
Labor	592	.649		.115	

Table A.2. *(cont.)*

Independent variables	N	Gross effect	R^2	Net effect	R^2
Peddlery	47	1.620		.784	
Other	160	-.094		.025	
Not ascertained	70	.976		-.360	
Size of place of residence			.011		.005
10,000+	1,603	-.209		-.129	
1,000 to 9,999	630	.136		.195	
Less than 1,000	519	.476		.161	
R^2 for total equation	2,752		.573		

Notes: The grand mean for NLC is 4.043. Gross effect coefficients are deviations of the category raw means from the grand mean; and the net effect coefficients, or regresstion coefficients, are the deviations of the category means from the grand mean net of the effects of the other explanatory variables. The gross effect R^2 is eta squared based on MCA, and the net effect R^2 is the squared multiple partial coefficient based on dummy variable regression.
*Less than 20 cases in base

Table A.3. *Gross and net effects of demographic, social, and economic variables on proportion of wives who had a live birth in 1970: Lebanon, 1971*

Independent variables	N	Gross effect	R^2	Net effect	R^2
Marriage duration (years)			.072		.083
0–4	442	.145		.167	
5–9	516	.117		.117	
10–14	636	.008		.011	
15–19	440	-.062		-.065	
20+	695	-.147		-.162	
Age at marriage (years)			.004		.010
12–16	572	.000		.020	
17–19	779	.020		.019	
20–21	477	.022		.021	
22–24	456	-.004		-.005	
25+	425	-.055		-.079	
Not ascertained	25	-.057		-.032	
Wife's education			.004		.002
No schooling	1,075	.016		.017	
Primary not completed	751	-.004		.000	

Table A.3. *(cont.)*

Independent variables	N	Gross effect	R^2	Net effect	R^2
Primary completed	385	.012		-.001	
Secondary not completed	279	-.002		-.003	
Secondary or higher completed	239	-.078		-.072	
Religion			.022		.012
Catholic	908	-.040		-.032	
Non-Catholic Christian	583	-.064		-.046	
Sunni	559	.043		.028	
Shi'a	560	.096		.080	
Druze	119	-.032		-.040	
Total family income (Lebanese pounds)			.011		.001
0–2,999	935	.037		.021	
3,000–5,999	750	.019		-.007	
6,000–9,999	332	-.036		-.019	
10,000–14,999	182	-.068		-.035	
15,000+	212	-.108		-.040	
Not ascertained	318	-.006		.019	
Husband's occupation			.011		.003
Professional/technical	119	-.107		-.037	
Business/management	457	-.343		-.156	
Clerical/sales	332	.000		.001	
Police/army/guard	169	.067		.032	
Crafts/operatives	554	.027		.016	
Farming	236	-.056		-.050	
Labor	590	.026		-.005	
Peddlery	47	.103		.047	
Other	157	-.019		-.004	
Not ascertained	68	-.070		.035	
Size of place of residence			.000		.000
10,000+	1,587	-.000		-.002	
1,000 to 9,999	624	-.007		.002	
less than 3,000	518	.009		.005	
R^2 for total equation	2,729		.105		

Note: The grand mean for this dependent variable is .217.

Table A.4. *Gross and net effects of demographic, social, and economic variables on ideal number of children reported: Lebanon, 1971*

Independent variables	N	Gross effect	R^2	Net effect	R^2
Marriage duration (years)			.038		.000 (.045)[a]
0–4	341	–.411		.112	
5–9	382	–.244		–.061	
10–14	463	–.024		–.102	
15–19	305	.236		–.006	
20+	474	.364		.072	
Age at marriage (years)			.005		.000
12–16	379	.142		–.101	
17–19	565	.006		–.064	
20–21	361	.009		.091	
22–24	339	–.009		.133	
25+	300	–.197		–.010	
Not ascertained	21	.074		–.011	
Parity			.097		.024
0	101	–.469		–.437	
1	201	–.591		–.549	
2	306	–.438		–.283	
3	309	–.356		–.222	
4	281	.001		.035	
5+	767	.534		.391	
Wife's education			.074		.017
No schooling	599	.487		.263	
Primary not completed	586	.043		.013	
Primary completed	330	–.177		–.027	
Secondary not completed	246	–.450		–.259	
Secondary or higher completed	204	–.724		–.453	
Religion			.056		.015
Catholic	664	–.039		–.028	
Non-Catholic Christian	457	–.300		–.143	
Sunni	390	–.102		–.066	
Shi'a	363	.681		.433	
Druze	91	–.491		–.528	
Total family income (Lebanese pounds)			.016		.003
0–2,999	540	.219		–.039	
3,000–5,999	559	.056		.026	
6,000–9,999	283	–.006		.102	

Table A.4. *(cont.)*

Independent variables	*N*	Gross effect	R^2	Net effect	R^2
10,000–14,999	161	-.334		-.016	
15,000+	195	-.286		.078	
Not ascertained	227	-.169		-.153	
Husband's occupation			.029		.016
Professional/technical	99	-.560		.023	
Business/management	365	.010		.143	
Clerical/sales	278	-.258		-.058	
Police/army/guard	126	-.003		-.086	
Crafts/operatives	434	-.034		-.030	
Farming	123	.563		.180	
Labor	361	.176		-.122	
Peddlery	27	-.270		-.533	
Other	115	.339		.338	
Not ascertained	37	-.379		-.461	
Size of place of residence			.022		.011
10,000+	1,249	-.123		-.081	
1,000 to 9,999	451	.030		.010	
Less than 1,000	265	.528		.366	
R^2 for total equation	1,965		.173		

Note: The grand mean for this dependent variable is 3.974.
[a]This is the squared multiple partial coefficient for marriage duration and parity; it represents the proportion of the variance explained in the dependent variable, ideal family size, by marriage duration and parity, after controlling for the other six independent variables.

Table A.5. *Gross and net effects of demographic, social, and economic variables on number of additional children wanted: Lebanon, 1971*

Independent variables	*N*	Gross effect	R^2	Net effect	R^2
Marriage duration (years)			.363		.072 (.313)[a]
0–4	380	1.540		.675	
5–9	433	.376		.318	
10–14	556	-.310		-.126	
15–19	388	-.494		-.251	
20+	639	-.601		-.354	

Table A.5. *(cont.)*

Independent variables	N	Gross effect	R^2	Net effect	R^2
Age at marriage (years)			.001		.001
12–16	491	–.217		–.010	
17–19	703	–.028		–.209	
20–21	413	.059		.009	
22–24	396	.082		.016	
25+	370	.184		.063	
Not ascertained	23	.064		–.100	
Parity			.381		.081
0	113	2.343		1.870	
1	226	1.291		.846	
2	339	.447		.229	
3	342	–.101		–.061	
4	340	–.351		–.253	
5+	1,036	–.535		–.383	
Wife's education			.016		.001
No schooling	856	–.115		.068	
Primary not completed	687	–.110		–.035	
Primary completed	365	.139		.030	
Secondary not completed	263	.270		.008	
Secondary or higher completed	225	.232		–.193	
Religion			.005		.022
Catholic	806	–.039		–.045	
Non-Catholic Christian	534	–.093		–.131	
Sunni	484	.005		.007	
Shi'a	468	.160		.239	
Druze	104	.012		–.085	
Total family income (Lebanese pounds)			.007		.001
0–2,999	758	.044		.074	
3,000–5,999	660	.077		.027	
6,000–9,999	318	–.042		–.040	
10,000–14,999	172	.090		–.057	
15,000+	204	–.106		–.142	
Not ascertained	284	–.232		–.079	
Husband's occupation			.006		.005
Professional/technical	113	.116		–.135	
Business/management	418	–.013		.090	
Clerical/sales	310	.101		–.080	

Table A.5. *(cont.)*

Independent variables	N	Gross effect	R^2	Net effect	R^2
Police/army/guard	145	.096		.017	
Crafts/operatives	506	-.013		.004	
Farming	181	-.083		.079	
Labor	486	-.027		-.023	
Peddlery	42	-.218		-.213	
Other	140	.103		.047	
Not ascertained	55	-.427		-.051	
Size of place of residence			.002		.005
10,000+	1,462	-.009		-.018	
1,000 to 9,999	551	-.084		-.038	
Less than 1,000	383	.085		.125	
R^2 for total equation	2,396		.463		

Note: The grand mean for this dependent variable is .718.
[a]This is the squared multiple partial coefficient for marriage duration and parity; it represents the proportion of the variance explained in the dependent variable, number of additional children wanted, by marriage duration and parity, after controlling for the other six independent variables.

Table A.6. *Gross and net effects of demographic, social, and economic variables on proportion of wives having knowledge of coitus interruptus: Lebanon, 1971*

Independent variables	N	Gross effect	R^2	Net effect	R^2
Marriage duration (years)			.007		.000 (.005)[a]
0–4	443	-.074		-.086	
5–9	517	.140		-.008	
10–14	636	.052		.042	
15–19	441	.009		.024	
20+	695	-.016		.007	
Age at marriage (years)			.004		.000
12–16	572	-.030		-.017	
17–19	779	-.008		-.011	
20–21	478	.038		.025	
22–24	458	.026		.021	
25+	420	-.024		-.019	
Not ascertained	25	.169		.176	

Table A.6. *(cont.)*

Independent variables	N	Gross effect	R^2	Net effect	R^2
Parity			.009		.002
0	184	−.126		−.103	
1	247	−.014		−.011	
2	368	.007		−.031	
3	386	.038		.004	
4	368	.075		.058	
5+	1,179	−.015		.009	
Wife's education X *religion*			.079		.033
No schooling:					
Catholic	264	−.135		−.058	
Non-Catholic Christian	122	−.185		−.131	
Sunni	272	−.010		−.061	
Shi'a	389	−.002		.049	
Druze	28	−.217		−.144	
Primary not completed:					
Catholic	276	−.050		−.047	
Non-Catholic Christian	186	−.119		−.102	
Sunni	133	.050		.107	
Shi'a	107	.261		.241	
Druze	51	−.215		−.131	
Primary completed:					
Catholic	167	.000		−.030	
Non-Catholic Christian	112	−.029		−.056	
Sunni	64	.194		.126	
Shi'a	29	.328		.325	
Druze	13	*		*	
Secondary not completed:					
Catholic	124	.021		−.054	
Non-Catholic Christian	82	.081		.008	
Sunni	43	.220		.171	
Shi'a	20	.369		.328	
Druze	11	*		*	
Secondary or higher completed:					
Catholic	79	.240		.123	
Non-Catholic Christian	82	.179		.058	
Sunni	47	.378		.250	
Shi'a	15	*		*	
Druze	16	*		*	

Table A.6. *(cont.)*

Independent variables	N	Gross effect	R^2	Net effect	R^2
Total family income (Lebanese pounds)			.064		.013
0–2,999	936	-.137		-.080	
3,000–5,999	750	.041		.034	
6,000–9,999	332	.102		.073	
10,000–14,999	183	.121		.045	
15,000+	212	.281		.169	
Not ascertained	319	-.058		-.058	
Husband's occupation			.051		.016
Professional/technical	119	.258		.104	
Business/management	458	.067		.002	
Clerical/sales	333	.140		.062	
Police/army/guard	169	-.011		-.036	
Crafts/operatives	554	.011		.024	
Farming	237	-.232		-.109	
Labor	590	-.075		-.006	
Peddlery	47	.059		.046	
Other	157	-.049		-.053	
Not ascertained	68	-.122		-.078	
Size of place of residence			.046		.021
10,000+	1,588	.085		.045	
1,000 to 9,999	626	-.065		-.021	
Less than 1,000	518	-.182		-.114	
R^2 for total equation	2,372		.154		

Note: The grand mean for this dependent variable is .431.
[a] This is the squared multiple partial coefficient for marriage duration and parity.
* Less than 20 cases in base.

Table A.7. *Gross and net effects of demographic, social, and economic variables on proportion of wives having knowledge of tubal ligation: Lebanon, 1971*

Independent variables	*N*	Gross effect	R^2	Net effect	R^2
Marriage duration (years)			.015		.010 (.010)[a]
0–4	443	.018		.077	
5–9	517	.061		.053	
10–14	636	.038		.020	
15–19	441	-.011		-.021	
20+	695	-.084		-.093	
Age at marriage (years)			.006		.006
12–16	572	-.031		.015	
17–19	779	.025		.030	
20–21	478	.033		.014	
22–24	458	.012		-.017	
25+	420	-.060		-.083	
Not ascertained	25	.061		.140	
Parity			.018		.004
0	184	-.097		-.204	
1	247	-.006		-.122	
2	368	.071		-.017	
3	386	.067		.013	
4	368	.060		.051	
5+	1,179	-.047		.043	
Wife's education × *religion*			.079		.034
No schooling:					
Catholic	264	-.129		-.041	
Non-Catholic Christian	122	-.099		-.039	
Sunni	272	-.139		-.125	
Shi'a	389	-.158		-.127	
Druze	28	.118		.175	
Primary not completed:					
Catholic	276	.033		.033	
Non-Catholic Christian	186	-.034		-.008	
Sunni	133	.081		.028	
Shi'a	107	.028		-.026	
Druze	51	.026		.064	
Primary completed:					
Catholic	167	.130		.095	
Non-Catholic Christian	112	.092		.070	
Sunni	64	.121		.034	
Shi'a	29	.158		.076	
Druze	13	*		*	

Table A.7. *(cont.)*

Independent variables	N	Gross effect	R^2	Net effect	R^2
Secondary not completed:					
Catholic	124	.157		.103	
Non-Catholic Christian	82	.066		.037	
Sunni	43	.238		.184	
Shi'a	20	.111		.017	
Druze	11	*		*	
Secondary or higher completed:					
Catholic	79	.122		.093	
Non-Catholic Christian	82	.200		.151	
Sunni	47	.176		.095	
Shi'a	15	*		*	
Druze	16	*		*	
Total family income (Lebanese pounds)			.058		.003
0–2,999	936	-.120		-.036	
3,000–5,999	750	.032		.013	
6,000–9,999	332	.150		.091	
10,000–14,999	183	.141		.057	
15,000+	212	.139		.035	
Not ascertained	319	-.052		-.076	
Husband's occupation			.066		.022
Professional/technical	119	.144		.033	
Business/management	458	.089		.042	
Clerical/sales	333	.099		.018	
Police/army/guard	169	.072		.020	
Crafts/operatives	554	.041		.026	
Farming	237	-.270		-.151	
Labor	590	-.095		-.021	
Peddlery	47	-.015		.041	
Other	157	.019		.018	
Not ascertained	68	-.121		-.049	
Size of place of residence			.040		.027
10,000+	1,588	.066		.041	
1,000 to 9,999	626	-.033		-.013	
Less than 1,000	518	-.161		-.109	
R^2 for total equation	2,732		.156		

Note: The grand mean for this dependent variable is .739.
[a]This is the squared multiple partial coefficient for marriage duration and parity.
*Less than 20 cases in base.

Table A.8. *Gross and net effects of demographic, social, and economic variables on proportion of wives who approve of contraception: Lebanon, 1971*

Independent variables	N	Gross effect	R^2	Net effect	R^2
Marriage duration (years)			.045		.000 (.041)[a]
0–4	443	–.207		.027	
5–9	517	.039		.016	
10–14	636	.097		.049	
15–19	441	.058		.030	
20+	695	–.022		–.038	
Age at marriage (years)			.007		.000
12–16	572	–.055		–.024	
17–19	779	.011		.010	
20–21	478	.031		.011	
22–24	458	.049		.023	
25+	420	–.027		–.027	
Not ascertained	25	–.107		.027	
Parity			.099		.029
0	184	–.493		–.511	
1	247	–.109		–.146	
2	368	.077		–.025	
3	386	.138		.033	
4	368	.091		.045	
5+	1,179	.002		.093	
Wife's education X religion			.132		.107
No schooling:					
Catholic	264	–.020		.036	
Non-Catholic Christian	122	–.110		–.086	
Sunni	272	–.219		–.197	
Shi'a	389	–.297		–.278	
Druze	28	.011		.062	
Primary not completed:					
Catholic	276	.104		.091	
Non-Catholic Christian	196	.048		.057	
Sunni	133	.077		.000	
Shi'a	107	.006		–.042	
Druze	51	–.020		.042	
Primary completed:					
Catholic	167	.189		.188	
Non-Catholic Christian	112	.110		.098	
Sunni	64	.130		.028	
Shi'a	29	.057		–.003	
Druze	13	*		*	

Table A.8. *(cont.)*

Independent variables	N	Gross effect	R^2	Net effect	R^2
Secondary not completed:					
Catholic	124	.212		.197	
Non-Catholic Christian	82	.211		.168	
Sunni	43	.123		.140	
Shi'a	20	.033		.024	
Druze	11	*		*	
Secondary or higher completed:					
Catholic	79	.193		.202	
Non-Catholic Christian	82	.161		.134	
Sunni	47	.205		.164	
Shi'a	15	*		*	
Druze	16	*		*	
Total family income (Lebanese pounds)			.086		.005
0–2,999	936	–.164		–.048	
3,000–5,999	750	.031		.025	
6,000–9,999	332	.185		.095	
10,000–14,999	183	.152		.044	
15,000+	212	.224		.064	
Not ascertained	319	–.022		–.085	
Husband's occupation			.076		.025
Professional/technical	119	.173		.056	
Business/management	458	.112		.041	
Clerical/sales	333	.126		.041	
Police/army/guard	169	–.005		–.066	
Crafts/operatives	554	.080		.050	
Farming	237	–.212		–.093	
Labor	590	–.162		–.053	
Peddlery	47	–.050		.070	
Other	157	.008		.009	
Not ascertained	68	–.153		–.104	
Size of place of residence			.041		.034
10,000+	1,588	.066		.051	
1,000 to 9,999	626	–.014		–.031	
Less than 1,000	518	–.185		–.119	
R^2 for total equation	2,732		.318		

Note: The grand mean for this dependent variable is .667.
[a]This is the squared multiple partial coefficient for marriage duration and parity.
*Less than 20 cases in base.

Table A.9. *Gross and net effects of demographic, social, and economic variables on proportion of wives who want to know more about family planning: Lebanon, 1971*

Independent variables	*N*	Gross effect	R^2	Net effect	R^2
Marriage duration (years)			.051		.059 (.063)[a]
0–4	446	.115		.027	
5–9	521	.093		.107	
10–14	639	.033		.016	
15–19	449	–.010		–.037	
20+	700	–.166		–.202	
Age at marriage (years)			.003		.012
12–16	575	–.015		.037	
17–19	786	.018		.026	
20–21	481	.012		–.006	
22–24	463	.026		–.004	
25+	425	–.055		–.093	
Not ascertained	25	.004		.104	
Parity			.014		.011
0	186	–.010		–.160	
1	250	.064		–.125	
2	371	.068		–.054	
3	391	.027		–.030	
4	372	.055		.056	
5+	1,185	.059		.060	
Wife's education			.040		.006
No schooling	1,077	–.114		–.067	
Primary not completed	761	.045		.031	
Primary completed	393	.080		.036	
Secondary not completed	283	.101		.063	
Secondary or higher completed	241	.116		.071	
Religion			.013		.014
Catholic	918	.001		.000	
Non-Catholic Christian	591	.031		.031	
Sunni	563	.054		.038	
Shi'a	564	–.096		–.078	
Druze	119	.038		.033	
Total family income (Lebanese pounds)			.018		.001
0–2,999	940	–.078		–.026	
3,000–5,999	754	.048		.037	
6,000–9,999	336	.068		.044	
10,000–14,999	185	.048		–.016	

Table A.9. *(cont.)*

Independent variables	N	Gross effect	R^2	Net effect	R^2
15,000+	212	.069		.015	
Not ascertained	328	-.027		.059	
Husband's occupation			.017		.003
Professional/technical	120	.082		.027	
Business/management	461	.059		.041	
Clerical/sales	337	.054		-.018	
Police/army/guard	172	.074		-.004	
Crafts/operatives	557	.015		-.016	
Farming	239	-.095		.020	
Labor	592	-.066		-.011	
Peddlery	47	-.017		.020	
Other	160	-.007		-.004	
Not ascertained	70	-.176		-.070	
Size of place of residence			.019		.011
10,000+	1,604	.042		.030	
1,000 to 9,999	632	-.007		.000	
Less than 1,000	519	-.121		-.093	
R^2 for total equation	2,755		.117		

Note: The grand mean for this dependent variable is .676.
[a]This is the squared multiple partial coefficient for marriage duration and parity.

Table A.10. *Gross and net effects of demographic, social, and economic variables on proportion of wives who ever used contraception: Lebanon, 1971*

Independent variables	N	Gross effect	R^2	Net effect	R^2
Marriage duration (years)			.026		.000 (.023)[a]
0–4	443	-.164		-.040	
5–9	517	.030		-.010	
10–14	636	.082		.042	
15–19	441	.041		.021	
20+	695	-.010		-.020	
Age at marriage (years)			.008		.000
12–16	572	-.049		-.017	
17–19	779	.003		.007	
20–21	478	.047		.029	

Table A.10. *(cont.)*

Independent variables	N	Gross effect	R^2	Net effect	R^2
22–24	458	.058		.030	
25+	420	-.051		-.056	
Not ascertained	25	-.099		.010	
Parity			.073		.014
0	184	-.422		-.422	
1	247	-.106		-.121	
2	368	.099		.036	
3	386	.139		.061	
4	368	.091		.055	
5+	1,179	-.017		.043	
Wife's education X *religion*			.103		.073
No schooling:					
Catholic	264	-.025		.015	
Non-Catholic Christian	122	-.089		-.076	
Sunni	272	-.204		-.178	
Shi'a	389	-.274		-.263	
Druze	28	.001		.024	
Primary not completed:					
Catholic	276	.139		.121	
Non-Catholic Christian	186	.061		.053	
Sunni	133	.043		-.010	
Shi'a	107	-.013		-.046	
Druze	51	-.008		.038	
Primary conpleted:					
Catholic	167	.160		.159	
Non-Catholic Christian	112	.010		.085	
Sunni	64	.158		.078	
Shi'a	29	.019		-.041	
Druze	13	*		*	
Secondary not completed:					
Catholic	124	.179		.170	
Non-Catholic Christian	82	.197		.154	
Sunni	43	.060		.080	
Shi'a	20	-.099		-.091	
Druze	11	*		*	
Secondary or higher completed:					
Catholic	79	.185		.216	
Non-Catholic Christian	82	.136		.129	
Sunni	47	.161		.142	
Shi'a	15	*		*	
Druze	16	*		*	

Table A.10. *(cont.)*

Independent variables	N	Gross effect	R^2	Net effect	R^2
Total family income (Lebanese pounds)			.056		.003
0–2,999	936	–.144		–.050	
3,000–5,999	750	.015		.013	
6,000–9,999	332	.176		.095	
10,000–14,999	183	.130		.045	
15,000+	212	.157		.028	
Not ascertained	319	.025		–.028	
Husband's occupation			.042		.007
Professional/technical	119	.107		–.003	
Business/management	458	.087		.019	
Clerical/sales	333	.111		.035	
Police/army/guard	169	.049		–.104	
Crafts/operatives	554	.065		.035	
Farming	237	–.165		–.068	
Labor	590	–.102		.005	
Peddlery	47	–.137		.009	
Other	157	.024		.024	
Not ascertained	68	–.219		–.171	
Size of place of residence			.017		.015
10,000+	1,588	.041		.031	
1,000 to 9,999	626	.008		–.012	
Less than 1,000	518	–.134		–.082	
R^2 for total equation	2,732		.217		

Note: The grand mean for this dependent variable is .533.
[a]This is the squared multiple partial coefficient for marriage duration and parity.

Table A.11. *Gross and net effects of demographic, social, and economic variables on proportion of wives currently contracepting: Lebanon, 1971*

Independent variables	*N*	Gross effect	R^2	Net effect	R^2
Marriage duration (years)			.007		.000 (.005)[a]
0–4	443	–.060		–.022	
5–9	517	.005		–.001	
10–14	636	.040		.023	
15–19	441	.027		.025	
20+	695	–.020		–.022	
Age at marriage (years)			.004		.001
12–16	572	–.046		–.011	
17–19	779	.012		.020	
20–21	478	.014		.001	
22–24	458	.012		–.014	
25+	420	.007		–.016	
Not ascertained	25	.082		.162	
Parity			.019		.004
0	184	–.135		–.157	
1	247	–.013		–.037	
2	368	.034		–.027	
3	386	.093		.031	
4	368	.028		–.001	
5+	1,179	–.026		.031	
Wife's education × *religion*			.140		.109
No schooling:					
Catholic	264	.020		.075	
Non-Catholic Christian	122	.087		.126	
Sunni	272	–.088		–.087	
Shi'a	389	–.310		–.286	
Druze	28	.059		.121	
Primary not completed:					
Catholic	176	.111		.114	
Non-Catholic Christian	186	.062		.060	
Sunni	133	.037		–.014	
Shi'a	107	–.172		–.181	
Druze	51	–.014		.043	
Primary completed:					
Catholic	167	.130		.122	
Non-Catholic Christian	112	.113		.086	
Sunni	64	.140		.076	
Shi'a	29	–.039		–.077	
Druze	13	*		*	

Table A.11. *(cont.)*

Independent variables	N	Gross effect	R^2	Net effect	R^2
Secondary not completed:					
Catholic	124	.138		.114	
Non-Catholic Christian	82	.153		.115	
Sunni	43	.063		.019	
Shi'a	20	.052		.019	
Druze	11	*		*	
Secondary or higher completed:					
Catholic	79	.126		.102	
Non-Catholic Christian	82	.104		.074	
Sunni	47	.117		.071	
Shi'a	15	*		*	
Druze	16	*		*	
Total family income (Lebanese pounds)			.053		.002
0–2,999	936	–.122		–.045	
3,000–5,999	750	.023		.014	
6,000–9,999	332	.103		.047	
10,000–14,999	183	.087		.011	
15,000+	212	.098		.006	
Not ascertained	319	.080		.041	
Husband's occupation			.047		.016
Professional/technical	119	.143		.068	
Business/management	458	.051		–.003	
Clerical/sales	333	.052		.006	
Police/army/guard	169	.084		.049	
Crafts/operatives	554	.047		.012	
Farming	237	–.144		–.051	
Labor	590	–.120		–.038	
Peddlery	47	.053		.154	
Other	157	.043		.033	
Not ascertained	68	–.033		–.017	
Size of place of residence			.037		.033
10,000+	1,588	.052		.045	
1,000 to 9,999	626	–.007		–.025	
Less than 1,000	518	–.151		–.109	
R^2 for total equation	2,732		.207		

Note: The grand mean for this dependent variable is .798.
[a]This is the squared multiple partial coefficient for marriage duration and parity.
*Less than 20 cases in base.

Table A.12. *Number of wives in sample by parity and wife's age*

	Wife's age								
Parity	15–19	20–24	25–29	30–34	35–39	40–44	45–49	Not ascertained	*N*
0	22	70	32	19	18	14	13	1	189
1	31	92	64	25	17	11	11	1	252
2	14	100	94	69	55	31	19	1	383
3	4	56	102	99	61	47	27		396
4		37	84	87	64	72	30		374
5		12	58	85	62	77	39		333
6		3	28	68	79	52	44		274
7		1	10	57	47	40	32		187
8		1	4	23	36	29	29		122
9		1	4	17	24	28	21		95
10		1	2	10	20	32	25	2	92
11				7	11	9	13		40
12			1		6	16	9		32
13					2	7	7		16
14					1	1	2		4
Not ascertained			3	1	1	1			6
Total	71	374	486	567	504	467	321	5	2,795

Table A.13. *Number of wives in sample by religion and wife's age*

	Wife's age								
Religion	15–19	20–24	25–29	30–34	35–39	40–44	45–49	Not ascertained	*N*
Catholic	19	102	163	188	177	170	105	1	925
Non-Catholic Christian	6	63	94	121	119	103	85	1	592
Sunni	21	98	107	102	100	81	54	1	564
Shi'a	20	88	95	125	82	93	63	1	567
Druze	5	19	20	26	20	18	11		119
Other		4	7	5	6	2	3	1	28
Total	71	374	486	567	504	467	321	5	2,795

Appendix B. Description of occupational categories

The occupational categories used in this study and examples for each category are given below. These particular categories were selected for two reasons. First, the descriptions of husband's occupation provided by the wives were short and not very detailed, therefore necessitating broad occupational groupings. Second, categories similar to those generally used in other nations were chosen so as to permit reasonable cross-national comparisons.

a. *Professional/technical:* Teachers, doctors, dentists, engineers, lab technicians, lawyers, editors, pharmacists (generally those with at least two years of college)

b. *Business/management:* Bankers and financial investors, insurance men, owners of businesses, (e.g., shops, stores)

c. *Clerical/sales:* Clerks in government or private industry, sales workers, typists, secretaries, bookkeepers

d. *Police/army/guard:* Watchmen, concierges, soldiers

e. *Crafts/operatives:* Metalworkers, machinists, plumbers, carpenters, mechanics, welders, drivers, shoemakers, weavers, repairmen

f. *Farming:* Gardeners, farmers (farm owners and tenants), dairy workers

g. *Labor:* Unskilled and semiskilled laborers, workers on construction and roads, sweepers, factory workers, fruit pickers, porters

h. *Peddlery:* Traveling peddlers for fruit, food, clothes, glass, and so forth

i. *Other:* Fishermen, teachers without college training (generally, jobs that do not fit categories above)

Appendix C. Questionnaire

Lebanon Family Planning Association

A sample study of family planning in Lebanon

House no. in the sample ____________________
District ____________________ Street ____________________
Town ____________________ House no. ____________________
Quarter ____________________ Floor ____________________
Apartment ____________________
Owner ____________________
Renter ____________________

First visit
Name of field-worker ____________________
Date of visit/ / /1971
Result of visit: Interview occurred ___ Interview did not occur ______
Reasons ____________________
Duration of interview ____________________ Minutes ______

Second visit
Name of field-worker ____________________
Date of visit/ / /1971
Result of visit: Amendment occurred ___ Amendment did not occur ___
Reasons ____________________
Duration of interview ____________________ Minutes ______

First precision: Accepted ___ Returned for more concise remarks ___ Signature of surveyor ______

Second precision: Accepted___ Returned for more concise remarks___ Signature of surveyor________

Signature of person concerned with symbols of card no. 1________________

Signature of person concerned with symbols of card no. 2 & 3________________

Signature of person checking up symbols of card no. 1________________

Signature of person checking up symbols of card no. 2 & 3________________

Remarks pertinent to the administration________________________

I. Information about housing accommodation and income

1. No. of rooms in the house (does not include kitchen and bathroom): ________________
2. Place of the bathroom:
   - private inside the house ________ 1
   - private outside the house ________ 2
   - shared inside the house ________ 3
   - shared outside the house ________ 4
   - does not exist ________ 5
3. Number of family members living permanently at home: ________________
4. Number of extra family members living permanently at home (does not include maids): ________________

In case of extra members:

5. Relationship to husband and wife: ____________ ________________
   ____________ ________________
   ____________ ________________
6. Condition of the house from inside (left to the judgment of the social worker):
   - deluxe _____ 1
   - above medium _____ 2
   - medium _____ 3
   - below medium _____ 4
   - bad condition _____ 5
7. Annual average income of members living permanently in the house (L.L.):
   - less than 1,500 L.L. _____ 1
   - 1,500 to less than 3,000 L.L. _____ 2

3,000 to less than 6,000 L.L.	____ 3
6,000 to less than 10,000 L.L.	____ 4
10,000 to less than 15,000 L.L.	____ 5
15,000 to less than 25,000 L.L.	____ 6
more than 25,000 L.L.	____ 7
no estimate given	____ 8
was not mentioned	____ 9

This section is left for the account of incomes:

Husband
Wife
Children
Income of extra members
Lands or agricultural products
Donations and miscellaneous aids

II. Social background of husband and wife

8. Date of birth of husband: ____________ ____________
month year

9. Religious sect:

Catholic	____ 1
non-Catholic	____ 2
Sunni	____ 3
Shi'a	____ 4
Druze	____ 5
Other sect	____ 6

10. Nationality:

Lebanese	____ 1
non-Lebanese	____ 2
Specify	____ 3

In case husband is a foreigner:

11. For how many hears has he been living in Lebanon? ____________
12. Date of birth of wife: ____________ ____________
month year
13. Religious sect of wife before marriage:

Catholic	____ 1
non-Catholic	____ 2
Sunni	____ 3
Shi'a	____ 4
Druze	____ 5
Other sect	____ 6

14. Nationality before marriage:

Lebanese	_____	1
non-Lebanese	_____	2
Specify	____________	3

15. Number of years wife worked before and after marriage:

	Before marriage	*After marriage*	
one year	______	______	1
two years	______	______	2
three years	______	______	3
four years	______	______	4
five years	______	______	5
six years	______	______	6
seven years	______	______	7
more than seven years no paid employment	______	______	8

16. Type of work:

	Husband	*Wife*
	____________	____________

17. Type of employment:

	Husband	Wife	
employed in a private sector	______	______	1
employed in a public sector	______	______	2
proprietor of work	______	______	3
self-employed	______	______	4

18. Nature of work:

permanent	______	______	1
seasonal	______	______	2
interrupted	______	______	3

19. Duration of time at work:

before noon	______	______	1
before and after noon	______	______	2
after noon	______	______	3
at night	______	______	4
not restricted to definite periods	______	______	5

20. Highest degree of education attained by him (or her):

illiterate	______	______	1
did not complete elementary education	______	______	2
completed elementary education	______	______	3

		Husband	*Wife*	
	did not complete secondary education	______	______	4
	completed secondary education	______	______	5
	did not complete university education	______	______	6
	completed university education	______	______	7
	does not know	______	______	8
21. Type of school in which he (or she) had followed up his (or her) education until secondary level:	governmental or public	______	______	1
	private religious	______	______	2
	private nonreligious	______	______	3
	governmental and private religious	______	______	4
	governmental and private nonreligious	______	______	5
	private religious and nonreligious	______	______	6
	governmental, private religious, and nonreligious	______	______	7
	did not attend any school	______	______	8
	does not know	______	______	9
22. Does he (or she) read newspapers or magazines?	not at all	______	______	1
	rarely	______	______	2
	occasionally	______	______	3
	constantly	______	______	4
23. Does he (or she) attend movies?	not at all	______	______	1
	rarely	______	______	2

		Husband	*Wife*	
	occasionally	______	______	3
	constantly	______	______	4
24. Activities or associations and clubs of which he (or she) is a member:	sports or athletic	______	______	1
	youth	______	______	2
	social & cultural	______	______	3
	religious	______	______	4
	familial	______	______	5
	political	______	______	6
	more than one activity	______	______	7
	is not a member of any association or club	______	______	8
	does not know	______	______	9

25. Relationship between them before marriage:	no relationship	____	1
	cousins	____	2
	distant relationship	____	3
26. Does the husband live with his wife constantly?	no	____	1
	yes	____	2
	other (specify)________________		
27. Number of marriages prior to husband's present marriage:	one	____	1
	two	____	2
	three	____	3
	four	____	4
	five or more	____	5
	was not married before	____	6
	does not know	____	7
28. Does he have another wife legally, at present?	has one extra wife	____	1

	has two extra wives	____ 2
	has three extra wives	____ 3
	does not have another wife	____ 4
	does not know	____ 5
29. Number of children from his other legal marriages, present and past:	one	____ 1
	two	____ 2
	three	____ 3
	four	____ 4
	five	____ 5
	six	____ 6
	seven or more	____ 7
	does not have any such children	____ 8
	does not know	____ 9

III. Some detailed social and medical information

30. Was the wife aware of any sexual matters before marriage? From what sources?	was not aware	____ 1
	knowledge through parents	____ 2
	knowledge through relatives & friends	____ 3
	knowledge from her doctor	____ 4
	knowledge from her readings	____ 5
	knowledge from more than one source	____ 6
31. Does she discuss sexual problems with her children?	Does not have children	____ 1
	children have not reached adolescence yet	____ 2
	discusses matters when asked to	____ 3
	does it on her own	____ 4

	does not discuss such problems with them	____	5
32. Does she discuss with her husband how they should bring their children up (health, diet, education, marriage)?	does not have children	____	1
	discusses it rarely	____	2
	discusses it occasionally	____	3
	discusses it frequently	____	4
	no discussion	____	5
33. What, in her own opinion, is the ideal number of children?	males	____	
	females	____	
	does not make any difference	____	
	no idea	____	
34. What, in her own opinion, should the space be between two deliveries?	one year	____	1
	two years	____	2
	three years	____	3
	four years	____	4
	five years or more	____	5
	does not make any difference	____	6
	no idea	____	7
35. Did she make any plans with her husband on the number of children wanted? and when?	made plans after the first child	____	1
	made plans after the second child	____	2
	made plans after the third child	____	3
	made plans after the fourth child	____	4
	made plans after the fifth or later	____	5
	made plans directly after marriage	____	6

Question	Response		Code
	did not make any plans ahead	____	7
	does not remember having made any plans	____	8
36. Does she desire to have more children? How many?	one	____	1
	two	____	2
	three	____	3
	four	____	4
	five	____	5
	does not wish to have any	____	6
	does not make any difference	____	7
37. After how many years of marriage did she desire to have her first child?	after one year	____	1
	after two years	____	2
	after three years	____	3
	after four years	____	4
	directly after marriage	____	5
	did not think about it	____	6
	did not make any difference with her	____	7
38. At what age did she have her menarche?	does not remember	____	
	at the age of	____	
39. Number of days between her menses:	does not know	____	
	irregular	____	
	number of days	____	
40. Nature of her menstrual period:	not painful	____	
	painful	____	
41. Has she had any gynecological operation? When?	has not had any	____	1
	yes, before marriage	____	2
	yes, after marriage	____	3
	yes, before and after marriage	____	4

IV. Information about contraceptive measures practiced

The answers to questions 42, 43, 44, 45, and 46 appear in the table on page 123.

42. The woman is asked to list the contraceptive methods she has heard about. (Field-worker puts an "X" in the appropriate box in column 1 for each method the woman mentions.)
43. Methods the woman did not mention are read to her, and she is asked to say whether or not she has heard about them. (Field-worker puts an "X" in the appropriate box in column 2 for every method the woman says she has heard about.)
44. The woman is asked if she knows how to practice the methods she mentioned or has heard about. (Field-worker puts an "X" in the appropriate box in column 3 for every method the woman knows how to practice.)
45. The woman is asked if she has ever practiced any of the methods she says she is familiar with. (Field-worker puts an "X" in the appropriate box in column 4 for every method the woman has practiced.)
46. The woman is asked if she is still practicing any of the methods she says she is familiar with. (Field-worker puts an "X" in the appropriate box in column 5 for every method the woman is still practicing.)
47. What is the wife's opinion, in general, of those women who use contraceptives? If she disapproves of such women, what are her reasons? If she approves, what are her reasons?

Disapproves:
for ethical reasons ____ 1
for religious reasons ____ 2
because of disapproval of birth control methods themselves ____ 3
other (specify) ____________
no idea ____________

Table for answers of questions no. 42, 43, 44, 45, and 46

Contraceptive devices	1 question no. 42	2 question no. 43	3 question no. 44	4 question no. 45	5 question no. 46
Rhythm					
Coitus interruptus					
Condom					
Oral pill					
Douching after intercourse					
Vaginal douche					
Cream					
Cervical cap					
IUD (loop)					
Sponge					
Vasectomy					
Tubal ligation					
Vaginal tablet, Aspro					
Other (specify)					

	Approves:		
	to preserve the family income	____	1
	to preserve the health of the mother	____	2
	to take care in the bringing up of each child	____	3
	to ensure child spacing and to reduce total number of births	____	4
	to devote woman's time to work	____	5
	to devote women's time to entertainment	____	6
	other (specify) ________________		
48. What is the attitude of her husband, in general, toward women using contraceptive measures?	disagree	____	1
	agree	____	2
	according to circumstances	____	3
	does not know	____	4
49. From what sources did she hear about contraception?	never heard of it	____	1
	from her husband	____	2
	from her parents	____	3
	from friends & relatives	____	4
	from a doctor	____	5
	from her own readings	____	6
	from more than one source	____	7
50. Does she have the interest to know more about contraception? From what sources?	does not desire to	____	1
	does not make any difference	____	2
	yes, through her husband	____	3
	yes, through her parents	____	4
	yes, through friends & relatives	____	5
	yes, through a doctor	____	6
	yes, through her own readings	____	7
	yes, from more than one source	____	8

51. When did she use contraception for the first time?

after her first baby	____	1
after her second baby	____	2
after her third baby	____	3
after her fourth baby	____	4
after her fifth baby or later	____	5
did not use it at all	____	6
does not remember	____	7
directly after marriage	____	8

52. Who made the decision to use contraception for the first time?

wife alone	____	1
husband alone	____	2
both agreed	____	3
not used	____	4
does not know	____	5

53. Did she get pregnant while using these contraceptive methods? Which method?

did not occur ____

occurred while using ____________

54. What is her attitude, and that of her husband, toward induced abortion?

	Husband	*Wife*	
disagree	______	______	1
agree	______	______	2
according to circumstances	______	______	3
no idea	______	______	4
does not know	______	______	5

V. Information about the deliveries of the wife

55. Date of her present marriage: ____________ ____________
month year

56. Was she married before?

married once	____	1
married twice	____	2

married three times	____	3
married four times or more	____	4
was not married before	____	5

57. Date of her first marriage: ____________ ____________
month year

58. Did she get pregnant during her previous marriages? ____________ ____________
no yes

If answer to question no. 58 was no, questionnaire was concluded.

59. Is she pregnant now? How advanced?

not pregnant	____	1
pregnant in her second month	____	2
pregnant in her third month	____	3
pregnant in her fourth month	____	4
pregnant in her fifth month	____	5
pregnant in her sixth month	____	6
pregnant in her seventh month	____	7
pregnant in her eighth month	____	8
pregnant in her ninth month	____	9
not sure of her dates	____	10

60. Number of children alive: ________
61. Number of children born alive but died later on: ________
62. Number of stillbirths: ________
63. Number of spontaneous abortions:
from pregnancies that did not exceed three months ________
from pregnancies that exceeded three months ________
64. Number of induced abortions: ________
65. Total number of pregnancies: ________
66. Number of premature deliveries: ________
67. Number of children born abnormal: ________
68. Number of deliveries according to the place where they occurred

(review questions no. 60, 61, 62):	maternity hospital	________
	home delivery performed by a doctor	________
	home delivery performed by a licensed midwife	________
	home delivery performed by a nonlicensed midwife	________
69. Number of induced abortions according to their results (review question no. 64):	safe	________
	bleeding	________
	others	________
70. Number of induced abortions according to the place of occurrence:	in a hospital, performed by a doctor	________
	in a clinic, performed by a doctor	________
	in a clinic, performed by a licensed midwife	________
	at home, performed by a doctor	________
	at home, performed by a licensed midwife	________
	at home, performed by a nonlicensed midwife	________

71. Number of induced abortions according to the

person by whom the decision was made:

wife alone	________
upon the request of husband	________
upon the request of doctor	________
with the consent of husband and wife	________

72. Children, dead and alive, born to the respondent during her marital life, by date of birth (review questions no. 60 and 61):

			Residence			
Child's first name	Month & year of birth	Sex	with his mother	not with his mother	Dead?	Age at death
1.						
2.						
3.						
4.						
5.						
6.						
7.						
8.						
9.						
10.						
11.						
12.						
13.						
14.						

Notes

Foreword

1 Makoto Nohara. "Social Determinants of Reproductive Behavior in Japan." Ph.D. dissertation, University of Michigan, 1980.
2 Central Bureau of Statistics of Indonesia and The World Fertility Survey. *Principal Report, Indonesia Fertility Survey, 1976.* Djakarta, 1978.

Chapter 2. Data and methodology

1 Evidence to support the survival differential argument comes from Khamis (1958), who found, in a special survey of villages with populations of over 1,000 in 1953, that the infant mortality rate was 195 for males and 315 for females. In contrast, our results indicate no reason to believe that there is a survival differential in favor of males. Separate analyses show that Lebanese mortality differentials appear to follow the general pattern of slightly higher survival rates for females (Chamie 1977a, p. 12).
2 Of course, the use of earlier data sets would considerably expand the observable portion of the pattern. However, in the case of Lebanon, the only available data comes from Yaukey's (1961) 1958 study, which, as is discussed later, is limited in a number of significant respects. Nevertheless, as is elaborated more fully in the final chapter, his results, when linked with those from the *NFFP* survey, strongly suggest the pattern depicted in Figure 2.

Chapter 3. Lebanese religious groups

1 The common practice in Lebanon is to classify the Druzes within the Muslim category. It is important to note, however, that the Druzes are doctrinally quite different from Sunnis, Shi'as, and other Muslim sects. Strictly speaking, therefore, on theological grounds it would not be correct to lump the Druzes together with the Sunnis and Shi'as. The Druzes should be treated as a distinct religious group.
2 The accuracy of the 1932 figures is by no means a settled matter. A number of groups maintain that there was an undercount of Lebanese Muslims because of the French practice of enumerating only those who were properly registered under Ottoman rule. It is argued that the French incorrectly excluded many Lebanese Muslims who had not registered themselves with the Turks in order that they might avoid Turkish military service, to which the Christians were not generally subject. The various estimates made since 1932 are also viewed as grossly inaccurate. Not only do they exclude many "Lebanese" Muslims who have not been able to obtain their citizenship, but the figures are also considered by many Muslim groups as being strongly biased in favor of certain Christian communities.
3 This percent, as well as those for the Greek Orthodox and Armenian Orthodox sects, is the average based on the figures in Table 1.

4 Details of Lebanon's history may be found in Hitti (1967), Hourani (1946), Khalaf (1979), and Salibi (1965).

5 According to Makarem (1974), Sunnis were so called after the Arabic word *sunna,* which, in the religious context, means the literal tradition of the Islamic custom and practice based on Mohammed's words and deeds; the Arabic word *shi'a* means "party," that is, the party of Ali, Mohammed's son-in-law.

6 For details, refer to Chevalier (1971), Mallat (1971), Courbage and Fargues (1973; 1974), Khalaf (1978a; 1978b; 1979), Smock and Smock (1975), and Tabbarah (1979).

7 Parts of this section are based on material that appeared earlier in Chamie (1976–77).

8 For further information, see Dib (1959) and Salem (1973).

9 Prior to the 1958 Lebanese civil conflict, governmental appointments were also made in the ratio of six Christians to five Muslims. After the conflict, however, the compromise worked out between the various warring factions stipulated that governmental appointments would be made according to the ratio of six Christians to six Muslims.

10 Restricting the calculations to women twenty-five years and older in order to avoid the problem of censoring does not alter the differentials in age at marriage, but only raises each of them by approximately half a year.

Chapter 4. Religious fertility differentials

1 Sunnis and Shi'as have lower survival rates than non-Catholic Christians, Catholics, and Druzes. Whereas Sunnis and Shi'as are consistently between 2 to 6 percent below the national averages, the others are from 1 to 5 percent above the averages.

2 As is the case in all such retrospective surveys, there are biases and problems of completeness and reliability. In the early stages of analysis, the data were compared to available external sources as well as internally checked. The results indicate that the data are of reasonably good quality. For example, the fertility rates from the *NFFP* survey are in agreement with expectations for Lebanon; the total fertility rate is approximately 4.5 births per woman, which is similar to other estimates for Lebanon (Courbage and Fargues 1973; Prothro and Diab 1974; République Libanaise, Ministère du Plan, 1970). Indirect population analysis techniques also provide estimates that indicate that births in the previous year were not underenumerated to any significant extent.

The results from a large number of checks for internal consistencies also indicated the soundness of the data. For example, in the following comparisons errors were nearly totally absent: total number of live births by number of living children plus children who died; number of abortions by number of pregnancies; the city size by district of residence; wife's age by marriage duration by age at marriage; women who ever used contraception by women currently contracepting; and ideal number of sons by ideal number of children.

The quality control that was maintained throughout the execution of the survey provides further confidence in the completeness of the data. For instance, there were a series of checks to ensure accurate and complete interviewing, such as reinterviewing a subsample of the sample. All of these checks indicated that the interviewers had done an exceptional job, and that the respondents were extremely cooperative and frank during the interviews. The low refusal rate (about 2 percent) is testimony not only to the hard work of the interviewers, but also to the high receptivity of the Lebanese couples.

3 It should be noted that the net deviations for number of children ever born and number of living children for the Sunnis and Shi'as follow this converging pattern except for those at the secondary not-completed level. Or, in other words, the differences in fertility between the Sunnis and Shi'as decrease as education increases except at the secondary not-completed level, where the differences are larger than at lower educational levels. Although it is difficult to say precisely why this occurred, we feel that it is most likely due to the small number (twenty) of Shi'as at this educational level.

Chapter 7. Summary and conclusions

1 For an explanatory discussion of the Lebanese civil war, see Chamie (1976-77), Salibi (1976), and Tabbarah (1979).

2 Another important demographic factor which is not discussed here is the presence of roughly 400,000 Palestinians in Lebanon, which has a resident population of about 2.5 million. Their presence has had a serious impact on the balance of power among the religio-political groups insofar as, for a variety of reasons, the Palestinians tend to align themselves to a great extent with the Muslim sects. For further information on this subject, see Salibi (1965, 1976), Hudson (1968), and Chamie 1976-77).

3 See Bogue (1971) for an explanation of the conversion of the total fertility rates into crude birthrates.

References

Abu-Khadra, Rihab. 1959. "Recent Changes in Lebanese Moslem Marriages Shown by Changes in Marriage Contracts." Master's thesis, American University of Beirut.

Abu-Lughod, Janet. 1965. "The Emergence of Differential Fertility in Urban Egypt." *Milbank Memorial Fund Quarterly* 43, part 2 (April):313–43.

Agwani, M. S. 1965. *The Lebanese Crisis, 1958: A Documentary Study.* Bombay: Asia Publishing House.

Aitken, Annie, and John Stoeckel. 1971. "Dynamics of the Muslim–Hindu Differential in Family Planning Practices in Rural East Pakistan." *Social Biology* 18(September):268–76.

Andrews, Frank M., James N. Morgan, John A. Sonquist, and Laura Klem. 1973. *Multiple Classification Analysis: A Report on a Computer Program for Multiple Regression Using Categorical Predictors.* Ann Arbor: University of Michigan, Survey Research Center.

Arowolo, Oladele Olawuyi. 1973. "Correlates of Fertility in Moslem Populations: An Empirical Analysis." Ph.D. dissertation, University of Pennsylvania.

Baaklini, Abdo I. 1976. *Legislative and Political Development: Lebanon, 1842–1972.* Durham, N.C.: Duke University Press, Consortium for Comparative Legislative Studies.

Baer, Gabriel. 1966. *Population and Society in the Arab East.* New York: Praeger.

Barakat, Halim. 1973. "Social and Political Integration in Lebanon: A Case of Social Mosaic." *Middle East Journal* 27(Summer):301–18.

Bean, Frank D., and Charles H. Wood. 1974. "Ethnic Variations in the Relationship between Income and Fertility." *Demography* 11(4):629–40.

Becker, Gary S. 1960. "An Economic Analysis of Fertility." In Coale, Ansley, ed., *Demographic and Economic Change in Developed Countries.* Princeton: Princeton University Press.

Blake, Judith, 1966. "The Americanization of Catholic Reproductive Ideals." *Population Studies* 20(July):27–43.

Bogue, Donald J. 1971. *Demographic Techniques of Fertility Analysis.* Chicago: University of Chicago, Community and Family Study Center.

Bongaarts, John. 1978. "A Framework for Analyzing the Proximate Determinants of Fertility." *Population and Development Review* 4(1):105–32.

Bouvier, Leon F. 1973. "The Fertility of Rhode Island Catholics: 1968–1969." *Sociological Analysis* 34(2):124–39.

Bouvier, Leon F., and S. L. N. Rao. 1975. *Socioreligious Factors in Fertility Decline.* Cambridge, Mass: Ballinger.

Brackbill, Yvonne, and Embry M. Howell. 1974. "Religious Differences in Family Size Among American Teenagers." *Sociological Analysis* 34(Spring):35–44.

Bumpass, Larry. 1969. "Age at Marriage as a Variable in Socioeconomic Differentials in Fertility." *Demography* 6(1):45–54.

Bumpass, Larry, and Charles F. Westoff. 1970. *The Later Years of Childbearing.* Princeton: Princeton University Press.

Burch, Thomas K. 1966. "The Fertility of North American Catholics: A Comparative Overview." *Demography* 3(1):174–81.

Busia, K. A. 1954. "Some Aspects of the Relation of Social Conditions to Human Fertility in the Gold Coast." In Lorimer, Frank, ed., *Culture and Human Fertility.* Switzerland: UNESCO:

Cairo Demographic Centre. 1970. *Demographic Measures and Population Growth in the Arab Countries.* Cairo:S.O.P. Press.

1971. *Fertility Trends and Differentials in Arab Countries.* Cairo:S.O.P. Press.

Caldwell, John C. 1968. "The Control of Family Size in Tropical Africa." *Demography* 5(2): 598–619.

Chamie, Joseph. 1976–77. "The Lebanese Civil War: An Investigation into the Causes." *World Affairs* 139(3):171–88.

1977a. "Religion and Population Dynamics in Lebanon." Ann Arbor (mimeographed).

1977b. "Religious Differentials in Fertility: Lebanon, 1971." *Population Studies* 31(2): 365–82.

1977c. "Religious Fertility Differentials: A Look at Some Hypotheses and Findings." *Population Bulletin of the United Nations Economic Commission for Western Asia* 13(July): 3–16.

Chevalier, Dominique. 1971. *La Société du Mont Liban à l'Epoque de la Révolution Industrielle en Europe.* Paris: Geuther, Librairie Orientalistic.

Chimali, Bisharah. 1915. "Mariage et Noces au Liban." *Antropos* X–XI:913–41.

Chou, Ru-Chi, and Susannah Brown. 1968. "A Comparison of the Size of Families of Roman Catholics and Non-Catholics in Great Britain." *Population Studies* 22:51–60.

Christopher, John. 1972. *The Islamic Tradition.* New York: Harper & Row.

Churchill, Charles. 1853. *Mont Lebanon, A Ten Years' Residence From 1842 to 1852.* London: Saunders and Otley.

Churchill, Charles W. 1954. *Beirut: A Socio-Economic Survey.* Beirut: Dar el-Kitab.

Churchill, Charles W., and Tony Sabbagh. 1968. "Beirut, Two-Time Levels, a Study of Development." *Middle East Economic Papers.* Beirut: American University of Beirut, Economic Research Institute.

Clark, Colin. 1967. *Population Growth and Land Use.* London: Macmillan.

Coale, Ansley. 1969. "The Decline of Fertility in Europe from the French Revolution to World War II." In Behrman, Samuel, Leslie Corsa, and Ronald Freedman, eds., *Fertility and Family Planning: A World View.* Ann Arbor: University of Michigan Press.

Coale, Ansley J., and Paul Demeny. 1966. *Regional Model Life Tables and Stable Populations.* Princeton: Princeton University Press.

Cooper, Charles, and Sydney S. Alexander. 1972. *Economic Development and Population Growth in the Middle East.* New York: Elsevier.

Courbage, Youssef, and Philippe Fargues. 1973. *La Situation Démographique au Liban, I: Mortalité, Fécondité et Projections, Méthodes et Résultats.* Beirut: Imprimerie Catholique.

1974. *La Situation Démographique au Liban, II: Analyse des Données.* Beirut: Imprimerie Catholique.

Crow, Ralph E. 1966. "Confessionalism, Public Administration and Efficiency in Lebanon." In Binder, Leonard, ed., *Politics in Lebanon.* New York: Wiley.

Cuinet, Vital. 1896. *Syrie, Liban et Palestine; géographie administrative, statistique et raisonnée.* Paris.

Davis, Kingsley. 1963. "The Theory of Change and Response in Modern Demographic History." *Population Index* 29(4):345–66.

Davis, Kinglsey, and Judith Blake. 1956. "Social Structure and Fertility: An Analytic Framework." *Economic Development and Cultural Change* 4(3):211–35.

Day, Lincoln H. 1964. "Fertility Differentials Among Catholics in Australia." *Milbank Memorial Fund Quarterly* 42, part 2(April):57–63.

1968. "Natality and Ethnocentrism: Some Relationships Suggested by an Analysis of Catholic–Protestant Differences." *Population Studies* 22(March):27–50.

De Jong, Gordon. 1965. "Religious Fundamentalism, Socio-Economic Status and Fertility Attitudes in the Southern Appalachians." *Demography* 2:540–8.

De Onis, Juan. 1975. "Ferocity of Lebanon's Strife Has Deep Roots in Religious and Class Fears." *New York Times* July 2.

Dib, George. 1959. "Selections from Riadh Solh's Speech in the Lebanese Assembly October 7, 1943) Embodying the Main Principles of the Lebanese 'National Pact.'" *Middle East Forum* 34(January):6–7.

1975. *Law and Population in Lebanon.* Law and Population Monograph Series Number 29. Medford, Mass.: Fletcher School of Law and Diplomacy.

Driver, Edwin D. 1963. *Differential Fertility in Central India.* Princeton: Princeton University Press.

El-Badry, M. A. 1965. "Trends in the Components of Population Growth in Arab Countries of the Middle East: A Survey of Present Information." *Demography* 2:140–86.

El-Hamamsy, Leila S. 1972. "Belief Systems and Family Planning in Peasant Societies." In Brown, H., and E. Hutchings, Jr., eds., *Are Our Descendants Doomed?* New York: Viking Press.

Epstein, Eliahu. 1946. "Demographic Problems of the Lebanon." *Journal of the Royal Asian Society* 33:150–4.

Fagley, Richard M. 1967. "Doctrines and Attitudes of Major Religions in Regard to Fertility." *Proceedings of the World Population Conference, Belgrade, 1965.* New York: United Nations.

Farsoun, Samih K. 1970. "Family Structure and Society in Modern Lebanon." In Sweet, Louise E., ed., *Peoples and Cultures of the Middle East.* Garden City. N.Y.: Natural History Press.

Fetter, George C. 1964. "A Comparative Study of Attitudes of Christian and of Moslem Lebanese Villages." *Journal for the Scientific Study of Religion* 4:48–59.

Fisher, Ronald A. 1958. *The Genetical Theory of Natural Selection.* New York: Dover.

Freedman, Ronald. 1967. "Applications of the Behavioral Sciences to Family Planning Programs." *Studies in Family Planning* 23(October):5–9.

Freedman, Ronald, and Larry Bumpass. 1966. "Fertility Expectations in the United States 1962–64." *Population Index* 32(2):181–97.

Freedman, Ronald, and John Y. Takeshita. 1969. *Family Planning in Taiwan.* Princeton: Princeton University Press.

Freedman, Ronald, Pascal Whelpton, and Arthur Campbell. 1959. *Family Planning, Sterility, and Population Growth.* New York: McGraw-Hill.

Freedman, Ronald, Pascal Whelpton, and John W. Smit. 1961. "Socio-Economic Factors in Religious Differentials in Fertility." *American Sociological Review* 26(August):608–14.

Fuller, Anne. 1961. *Buarij: Portrait of a Lebanese Muslim Village.* Cambridge, Mass.: Harvard University Press, Harvard Middle Eastern Monographs.

Gibb, Sir Alexander, et al. 1948. *The Economic Development of Lebanon.* London: Gibb and Partners.

Glass, David V. 1968. "Fertility Trends in Europe since the Second World War." *Population Studies* 22(March):103–46.

Goldberg, David. 1959. "The Fertility of Two-Generation Urbanites." *Population Studies* 12(March):214–22.

1965. "Fertility and Fertility Differentials: Some Observations on Recent Changes in the United States." In Sheps, Mindel C., and Jeanne Clare Ridley, eds., *Public Health and Population Change.* Pittsburgh: University of Pittsburgh Press.

Goldberger, Arthur. 1964. *Econometric Theory.* New York: Wiley.

Goldscheider, Calvin. 1971. *Population, Modernization and Social Structure.* Boston: Little, Brown.

Goldscheider, Calvin, and P. R. Uhlenberg. 1969. "Minority Group Status and Fertility." *American Journal of Sociology* 74(4):361-72.

Goldstein, Sidney. 1970. "Religious Fertility Differentials in Thailand, 1960." *Population Studies* 24(November):325-37.

Goode, William, 1963. *World Revolution and Family Patterns.* New York: Free Press.

Goodman, Leo. 1973. "Causal Analysis of Data from Panel Studies and Other Kinds of Surveys." *American Journal of Sociology* 78(March):1135-91.

Greig, James D. 1973. "Mauritius: Religion and Population Pressure." In Smith, T. E., ed., *The Politics of Family Planning in the Third World.* London: Allen & Unwin.

Guillaume, Alfred. 1956. *Islam.* Baltimore: Penguin Books.

Gulick, John. 1955. *Social Structure and Culture Change in a Lebanese Village.* New York: Wenner-Gren Foundation.

1967. *Tripoli: A Modern Arab City.* Cambridge, Mass.: Harvard University Press.

Haddad, George. 1950. *Fifty Years of Modern Syria and Lebanon.* Beirut: Dar-al-Hayat.

Harfouche, Jamal Karam. 1965. *Social Structure of Low-Income Families in Lebanon.* Beirut: Khayat.

Harik, Iliya F. 1968. *Politics and Change in a Traditional Society: Lebanon, 1711-1845.* Princeton: Princeton University Press.

Hastings, Donald, et al. 1972. "Mormonisms and Birth Planning: The Discrepancy between Church Authorities' Teachings and Lay Attitudes." *Population Studies* 26(1):19-28.

Hawthorn, Geoffrey. 1970. *The Sociology of Fertility.* London: Collier-Macmillan.

Higgins, Edward. 1964. "Differential Fertility Outlook and Patterns among Major Religious Groups in Johannesburg." *Social Compass* 11(1):23-62.

Himadeh, S. B. 1936. *Economic Organization of Syria.* Beirut: Khayat.

Hitti, Philip. 1967. *Lebanon in History.* New York: St. Martin's Press.

Holler, Joanne E. 1964. *Population Growth and Social Change in the Middle East.* Washington, D.C.: George Washington University, Population Research Project.

Hourani, Albert H. 1946. *Syria and Lebanon.* London: Oxford University Press.

Hudson, Michael C. 1968. *The Precarious Republic - Political Modernization in Lebanon.* New York: Random House.

Hurewitz, J. C. 1966. "Lebanese Democracy in Its International Setting." In Binder, Leonard, ed., *Politics in Lebanon.* New York: Wiley.

Jones, Gavin, and Dorothy Nortman. 1968. "Roman Catholic Fertility and Family Planning: A Comparative Review of the Research Literature." *Studies in Family Planning* 34(October): 1-27.

Kennedy, Robert E., Jr. 1973. "Minority Group Status and Fertility: The Irish." *American Sociological Review* 38(February):85-96.

Kewenig, Wilhem. 1965. *Die Koexistenz der Religions-gemeinschaften in Libanon.* Berlin: Walter De Gruyter.

Khalaf, Samir. 1968. "Primordial Ties and Politics in Lebanon." *Middle Eastern Studies* 4(April):243-69.

1972. "Adaptive Modernization: The Case for Lebanon." In Cooper, Charles, and Sidney Alexander, eds., *Economic Development and Population Growth in the Middle East.* New York: Elsevier.

1978a. "Population and Family Planning in Lebanon: Problems, Perceptions and Programs." Paper submitted to Research and Training Project on Cultural Values and Population Policy, Institute of Society, Ethics and the Life Sciences, Hastings, N.Y. May (mimeographed).

1978b. "Communal Conflict in 19th Century Lebanon." Paper presented at Princeton Millet Conference, June 12-15 (mimeographed).

1979. *Persistence and Change in 19th Century Lebanon.* Beirut: American University of Beirut Press.

Khamis, Salem H. 1958. "A Report on a Pilot Infant Mortality Survey of Rural Lebanon." *Proceedings of the Thirteenth Session of the International Statistics Institute, 1957.* Stockholm.

Khuri, Fuad. 1967. "A Comparative Study of Migration Patterns in Two Lebanese Villages." *Human Organization* 26(4):206–12.

1975. *From Village to Suburb: Order and Change in Greater Beirut.* Chicago: University of Chicago Press.

Kirk, Dudley. 1967. "Factors Affecting Moslem Natality." *Proceedings of the World Population Conference, Belgrade, 1965.* New York: United Nations.

Knodel, John E. 1974. *The Decline of Fertility in Germany, 1871–1939.* Princeton: Princeton University Press.

Krotki, Karol, and Evelyn Lapierre. 1968. "La Fecondité au Canada la Religion, l'Origine Ethnique, et l'Etat Matrimonial." *Population* 23:815–34.

Lazerwitz, Bernard. 1970. "The Association between Religio-Ethnic Identification and Fertility among 'Contemporary' Protestants and Jews." *Sociological Quarterly* 2(Summer):307–20.

Lebanon Family Planning Association. 1974. *The Family in Lebanon (in Arabic).* Beirut: Lebanon Family Planning Association.

Lenski, Gerhard. 1961. *The Religious Factor.* New York: Doubleday/Anchor Books.

Lerner, Daniel. 1958. *The Passing of Traditional Society.* Glencoe, Ill.: Free Press.

Long, Larry H. 1970. "Fertility Patterns among Religious Groups in Canada." *Demography* 7(2):135–49.

Longrigg, Stephen H. 1958. *Syria and Lebanon Under French Mandate.* New York: Oxford University Press.

Makarem, Sami Nasib. 1974. *The Druze Faith.* Delmar, N.Y.: Caravan Books.

Mallat, Hyam. 1971. L'amengement du Territoire en de L'environment au Liban, Analyse Economique et Sociale. *Beirut: Imprime par Dar Ghandour.*

Mallat, Raymond A. 1973. *70 Years of Money Muddling in Lebanon, 1900–1970.* Beirut: Aleph Publishers.

Mandelbaum, David G. 1974. *Human Fertility in India.* Berkeley: University of California Press.

Markham, James M. 1975. "In Embattled Beirut, Nerves Are Taut and the Future Is Uncertain." *New York Times,* July 19.

Matras, Judah. 1973. "On Changing Matchmaking, Marriage, and Fertility in Israel: Some Findings, Problems, and Hypotheses." *American Journal of Sociology* 79(September): 364–87.

Mayer, Albert J., and Sue Marx. 1957. "Social Change, Religion, and Birth Rates." *American Journal of Sociology* 62(January):383–90.

Mazur, Peter D. 1967. "Fertility among Ethnic Groups in the USSR." *Demography* 4(1): 172–95.

Mazure, Claude. 1964. *Demographie-Liban et Perspective.* Beirut: Ministry of Planning.

Mekkawi, M. M. 1970. *The Population of Lebanon.* Beirut (mimeographed).

Meo, Leila M. T. 1965. *Lebanon: Improbable Nation.* Bloomington: Indiana University Press.

Milne, Robin G. 1973. "Family Planning in Malta." *Population Studies* 27(2):373–86.

Moore, Maurice J. 1973. *Death of a Dogma? The American Catholic Clergy's Views of Contraception.* Chicago: University of Chicago, Community and Family Study Center.

Moors, H. G. 1978. *The Netherlands Survey on Fertility and Parenthood Motivation, 1975: A Summary of Findings.* World Fertility Survey No. 12. Voorburg, Netherlands: International Statistical Institute.

Morgan, James, John A. Sonquist, and Elizabeth Baker. 1971. *Searching for Structure.* Ann Arbor: University of Michigan, Institute for Social Research.

Mroueh, Adnan. 1974. "The Population Explosion: Urgent Need for Control and Planning." *The Arab Economist* (September):13.

Nakib, Khalil A. 1972. "Bureaucracy and Development: A Study of the Lebanese Civil Service." Ph.D. dissertation, Florida State University.

Nazer, Isam R., ed. 1972. *Induced Abortion: A Hazard to Public Health?* Beirut: Aleph Publishers.

ed. 1974. *Islam and Family Planning.* Beirut: Imprimerie Catholique.

Nerlove, Marc, and S. James Press. 1973. *Univariate and Multivariate Log-Linear and Logistic Models.* Santa Monica, Calif.: Rand Corporation.

Nixon, J. W. 1963. "Some Demographic Characteristics of Protestants and Catholics in Switzerland." *International Population Conference, 1961.* No. 2. New York.

Noonan, John T., Jr. 1965. *Contraception: A History of Its Treatment by Catholic Theologians and Canonists.* Cambridge, Mass.: Harvard University Press.

Omran, Abdel R. 1973. "Islam and Fertility Control." In Omran, Abdel R., ed., *Egypt: Population Problems and Prospects.* Chapel Hill: University of North Carolina, Carolina Population Center.

Paul VI. 1968. *Humanae Vitae.* July 25. (Full translation into English in *National Catholic Reporter,* August 17, 1968).

Petersen, William. 1969. *Population.* 2nd edition. London: Macmillan.

Pitcher, Brian, et al. 1974. "Residency Differentials in Mormon Fertility." *Population Studies* 28(1):143–51.

Pius XII. 1958. "The Large Family." *The Pope Speaks* 4(Spring):363–4.

Polk, William. 1963. *The Opening of Southern Lebanon, 1788–1840.* Cambridge, Mass.: Harvard University Press.

Population Council. 1970. *A Manual for Surveys of Fertility and Family Planning: Knowledge, Attitudes and Practices.* New York: The Population Council.

Prothro, Edwin Terry, and Lutfy Najib Diab. 1974. *Changing Family Patterns in the Arab East.* Beirut: Heidelberg Press.

Qubain, Fahim I. 1961. *Crisis in Lebanon.* Washington, D.C.: The Middle East Institute.

République Libanaise, Ministère du Plan. 1960. *Besoins et Possibilités de Developments du Liban.* Vols I, II, and Appendixes.

Ministère du Plan, Service des Activites Regionales. 1967. *La Population du Liban: Enquete par Sondage, 1964.*

Ministère de la Santé. 1970. *Rapport Annuel des Statistiques Sanitaires.*

Ministère du Plan. 1970. *Recueil de Statistiques Libanaises.* Vol. 6. Direction Centrale de la Statistique.

Direction Centrale de la Statistique. 1972. *L'Enquête par Sondage sur la Population Active au Liban.*

Ritchey, P. Neal. 1975. "The Effect of Minority Group Status on Fertility: A Re-examination of Concepts." *Population Studies* 29(2):249–57.

Rizk, Hanna. 1963. "Social and Psychological Factors Affecting Fertility in the United Arab Republic." *Marriage and Family Living* 25(1):69–73.

1973. "National Fertility Sample Survey for Jordan, 1972: The Study and Some Findings." *Population Bulletin* (UNESOB) 5(July):14–31.

Roberts, Robert E., and Eun Sul Lee. 1974. "Minority Group Status and Fertility Revisited." *American Journal of Sociology* 80(September):503–23.

Rosten, Leo. 1975. *Religions of America.* New York: Simon & Schuster.

Ryder, Norman. 1973. "Recent Trends and Group Differences in Fertility." In Westoff,

Charles F., ed., *Toward the End of Growth.* Englewood Cliffs, N.J.: Prentice-Hall.

Ryder, Norman B., and Charles F. Westoff. 1971. *Reproduction in the U.S.: 1965.* Princeton: Princeton University Press.

Sabagh, Georges. 1970. "The Demography of the Middle East." *Middle East Studies Association Bulletin* 4(2):1–19.

Safa, Elie. 1960. *L'Emigration Libanaise.* Beirut: University of St. Joseph.

Sahlins, Marshall, and Elman Service. 1960. *Evolution and Culture.* Ann Arbor: University of Michigan Press.

Saleh, S. 1972. "Women in Islam: Their Status in Religion and Traditional Culture." *International Journal of Sociology of the Family* 2:1–8.

Salem, Elie Adib. 1973. *Modernization without Revolution: Lebanon's Experience.* Bloomington: Indiana University Press.

Salibi, Kamal S. 1965. *The Modern History of Lebanon.* London: Weidenfeld and Nicholson.

1976. *Crossroads to Civil War: Lebanon, 1958–1976.* Delmar: Caravan Books.

Salwa C. Nasser Foundation. 1969. *Cultural Resources in Lebanon.* Beirut: Librairie du Liban.

Saouda, Youssef. 1919. *Pour le Liban.* Beirut.

Schieffelin, Olivia. 1967. *Muslim Attitudes toward Family Planning.* New York: The Population Council.

Schultz, T. Paul. 1972. "Fertility Patterns and Their Determinants in the Arab Middle East." In Cooper, Charles A., and Sidney S. Alexander, eds., *Economic Development and Population Growth in the Middle East.* New York: Elsevier.

Schwarz, Karl. 1965. "Nombre d'Enfants suivant le Milieu Physique et Social en Allemagne Occidentals." *Population* 20(1):72–92.

Shryock, Henry S., and Jacob S. Siegal. 1973. *The Methods and Materials of Demography.* Washington, D.C.: Government Printing Office.

Sinha, J. N. 1957. "Differential Fertility and Family Limitation in an Urban Community of Uttar Pradesh." *Population Studies* 11(November):157–69.

Sly, David F. 1970. "Minority Group Status and Fertility: An Extension of Goldscheider and Uhlenberg." *American Journal of Sociology* 76(November):443–59.

Smit, John William. 1964. "A Matched Group Study of Religious Differentials in Fertility and Family Planning." Ph.D. dissertation, University of Michigan.

Smock, David R., and Audrey C. Smock. 1975. *The Politics of Pluralism: A Comparative Study of Lebanon and Ghana.* New York: Elsevier.

Spicer, Judith C., and Susan O. Gustavus. 1974. "Mormon Fertility through Half a Century: Another Test of the Americanization Hypothesis." *Social Biology* 21(1):70–6.

Stouffer, Samuel. 1935 "Trends in the Fertility of Catholics and Non-Catholics." *American Journal of Sociology* 4(September):143–54.

Suits, Daniel. 1957. "The Use of Dummy Variables in Regression Equations." *Journal of the American Statistical Association* 52:548–51.

Sweet, Louise E. 1970. *Peoples and Cultures of the Middle East.* New York: Natural History Press.

Tabbarah, Bahige B. 1954. "Les Forces Politiques Actuelles au Liban." Ph.D. dissertation, University of Grenoble.

Tabbarah, Riad B. 1979. "Background to the Lebanese Conflict." *International Journal of Comparative Sociology* XX(1–2):101–21.

Taeuber, Irene B. 1955. "Cyprus: The Demography of a Strategic Island." *Population Index* 21(1):4–20.

Tanas, Raja. 1974. "Family Planning Knowledge, Attitudes and Practices in Tyre, Lebanon." Master's thesis, American University of Beirut.

Tannous, Afif I. 1942. "Emigration, a Force of Social Change in an Arab Village." *Rural Sociology* VII(March):63–6.

Thorne, Melvyn C., and Joel Montague. 1973. "Special Characteristics of Population Policy in the Middle East and North Africa." *International Journal of Health Services* 3(4):779–90.

Touma, Toufic. 1958. *Un Village de Montagne au Liban.* Paris: Mouton.

Trotsky, Leon. n.d. *The History of the Russian Revolution.* Ann Arbor: University of Michigan Press.

United Nations. 1969. *Manual IV: Methods of Estimating Basic Demographic Measures from Incomplete Data.* Population Studies No. 42. New York: United Nations.

1970. *Variables and Questionnaires for Comparative Fertility Surveys.* Population Studies No. 45, New York: United Nations.

1972. "Some Demographic Characteristics of Women Having Delivered at the Maternity Clinic of Baabda Hospital (Suburbs of Beirut) in 1968." *Population Bulletin of the United Nations Economic and Social Office in Beirut.* July.

1972. "Survey of the Economically Active Population in Lebanon, 1970: Methodology and Results." *Population Bulletin of the United Nations Economic and Social Office in Beirut.* July.

1973. "Demographic Characteristics of Beirut City in 1970." *Population Bulletin of the United Nations Economic and Social Office in Beirut.* July.

1973. *Determinants and Consequences of Population Trends.* New York: United Nations.

Valsecchi, Ambrogio. 1968. *Controversy: The Birth Control Debate 1958–68.* Washington, D.C.: Corpus Books.

Van Dusen, Roxan. 1973. "Social Changes and Decision Making: Family Planning in Lebanon." Ph.D. dissertation, Johns Hopkins University.

Van Heek, F. 1956. "Roman-Catholicism and Fertility in the Netherlands." *Population Studies* 10(2):125–38.

Van Praag, Philip, and Louis Lohle-Tart. 1974. "The Netherlands." In Berelson, Bernard, ed., *Population Policy in Developed Countries.* New York: McGraw-Hill.

Visaria, Leela. 1974. "Religious Differentials in Fertility." In Bose, Ashish, et al., eds. *Population in India's Development 1947–2000.* New Delhi: Vikas.

Wall, Michael. 1974. "The Tightrope Country, A Survey of Lebanon." *The Economist:* January 26 (supplement).

Ware, Helen. 1974. "Ideal Family Size." *Occasional Paper No. 13.* World Fertility Survey. Voorburg, Netherlands: International Statistical Institute.

Weiner, Myron. 1970. *Perceptions of Population Change in India: A Field Report.* Cambridge, Mass.: Massachusetts Institute of Technology, Center for International Studies.

Westoff, Charles F. 1959. "Religion and Fertility in Metropolitan America." In *Thirty Years of Research in Human Fertility: Retrospect and Prospect.* Annual Conference of Milbank Memorial Fund, October 22–3, 1958. New York: Milbank Memorial Fund.

Westoff, Charles F., and Larry Bumpass. 1973. "The Revolution in Birth Control Practices of U.S. Roman Catholics." *Science:* (January 5):41–4.

Westoff, Charles F., and Elise F. Jones. 1977. "The Secularization of U.S. Catholic Birth Control Practices." *Family Planning Perspectives* 9:203–7.

1978. "The End of 'Catholic' Fertility." Paper presented at Population Association of America, Atlanta, Ga., April 12–15 (revised October 16, 1978; mimeographed).

Westoff, Charles F., and Raymond H. Potvin. 1967. *College Women and Fertility Values.* Princeton: Princeton University Press.

Westoff, Charles F., and Norman B. Ryder. 1969. "Recent Trends in Attitudes toward Fertility Control and the Practice of Contraception in the U.S." In Behrman, Samuel, Ronald Freedman, and Leslie Corsa, eds., *Fertility and Family Planning.* Ann Arbor: University of Michigan Press.

Whelpton, Pascal K., Arthur A. Campbell, and J. E. Patterson. 1966. *Fertility and Family Planning in the United States.* Princeton: Princeton University Press.

World Bank. 1974. *Population Policies and Economic Development.* Baltimore: Johns Hopkins University Press.

World Health Organization. 1976. *Family Formation Patterns and Health: An International Collaborative Study in India, Iran, Lebanon, Philippines, and Turkey.* Geneva: WHO.

Yaukey, David. 1961. *Fertility Differences in a Modernizing Country: A Survey of Lebanese Couples.* Princeton: Princeton University Press.

Zimmer, Basil, and Calvin Goldscheider. 1966. "A Further Look at Catholic Fertility." *Demography* 3(2):462–9.

Ziyadeh, Nicola A. 1957. *Syria and Lebanon.* London: Ernest Benn.

Zurayk, Huda. 1977. "Sources of Demographic Data in Lebanon." *Population Bulletin of the United Nations Economic Commission for Western Asia* 12(January):27–33.

1977. "The Effect of Education of Women and Urbanization on Actual and Desired Fertility and on Fertility Control in Lebanon." *Population Bulletin of the United Nations Economic Commission for Western Asia* 13(July):32–41.

Zuwiyya-Yamak, Labib. 1966. *The Syrian Social Nationalist Party: An Ideological Analysis.* Cambridge, Mass: Harvard University Press.

السكّان (كارتفاع نسبة المهاجرين المسيحيين الى الخارج) وعدم وجود تغيرات مماثلة لها في التوزيع السياسي والحكومي للسلطة قد ساعد على العنف السائد في البلاد حاليا. فاذا كان لبنان أو غيره من المجتمعات ذات الديانات المتعددة يرغب بمواصلة العمل ضمن نظام حكومي طائفي ، يعتمد على التمثيل النسبي لهذه الطوائف ، فمن الصواب أن يأخذ بالاعتبار التغييرات الديموغرافية الكبيرة في التركيب الديني للسكّان ، وان تسوى هذه التغييرات ضمن التنظيمات الحكومية والسياسية على نحو معتدل. وما عدا ذلك سيقود الوضع حتما الى مزيد من العداء والفشل والعنف.

الوسائل المشجعة على تنظيم الأسرة ، كلها أمور سوف يكون لها دور ايجابي في التحكم بموضوع الخصوبة .

ان النتائج المشار اليها انفا ذات أهمية قصوى لدى المسؤولين عن اتخاذ القرارات السكانية في تلك الدول التي يكون للمعتقد الديني حساسية خاصة وذلك لاعتبارات عديدة . فعلى متخذى القرارات أولا ادراك دور المعتقد الديني في اختلافات الخصوبة ، ولكن بشرط ان يكون ذلك في نطاق مستويات اجتماعية واقتصادية معينة . كما عليهم ثانيا الادراك بأن تقليص الاختلافات الدينية الكبيرة والمتعلقة بالخصوبة يمكن ان يتحقق عن طريق الارتقاء بالمستويات المعيشية الاجتماعية والاقتصادية للسكان . حيث سيؤدى عدم الارتقاء هذا الى أحداث مفجعة ، على النظام السياسي والاستقرار عامة .

وأخيرا ، فقد يكون من أبرز ما توصل اليه هذا البحث هو مدى الاعتماد على الافتراضات التفاعلية في تفسير الاختلافات الدينية خارج لبنان . وبالرغم من أن الاجابة الدقيقة على هذا السؤال تستلزم توافر بيانات وافية تأخذ بالحسبان المتغيرات الديموغرافية والاجتماعية والاقتصادية للنواحي الدينية السائدة ، فان الابحاث سوف تسهم في تأكيد ان الافتراضات التفاعلية قابلة للتعميم على الدول المختلفة .

وفي الختام ، وبالرغم من ان هذا البحث لم يتطرق بشكل عام الى الاحداث المفجعة التي يمر بها لبنان ، فان نتائجه لا يمكن الا أن تتعلق بالصراع الدائر على الساحة اللبنانية . فالفوارق الكبيرة في الانجاب بين الطوائف الدينية كانت وستظل ذات تأثير بالغ على استقرار النظام الاجتماعي والسياسي في البلاد .

عندما انشأت فرنسا دولة لبنان الكبير عام ١٩٢٠ ، أصبح التوزيع العددى للطوائف الدينية بين سكان لبنان قضية خطيرة وقابلة للاشتعال . ووفقا للدستور اللبناني فان مجلس النواب اللبناني ينتخب من السكان ، بحيث تتمثل فيه النسب المختلفة للطوائف الدينية . وفوارق نسب الخصوبة القائمة بين المذاهب الدينية يقابلها تغييرات في التركيب السكاني ، الأمر الذى يحقق بدوره ضغوطا في توزيع السلطة القائمة بين المجتمعات الدينية .

ولعل من المتفق عليه حاليا ان المسلمين يشكلون غالبية الشعب اللبناني ، وبالنظر للفوارق الكبيرة في نسب الخصوبة القائمة بين مختلف الطوائف ، فانه من المعتقد ان حجم السكان المسلمين سيستمر في الزيادة . وبالاضافة الى ذلك ، فمعظم المراقبين يسلمون بأن التوزيع النسبي للطوائف بين السكان قد تغير بلا شك منذ سنة ١٩٣٢ . فمثلا ، من المحتمل ان تكون الطائفة الشيعية الان أكبر طائفة ، وان لم تكن هي الطائفة الكبرى حاليا فانها ستصبح كذلك في المستقبل القريب اذا افترضنا ان نسب الخصوبة الحالية ستستمر دون تغييرات جوهرية في الوفيات والهجرة . وكذلك الطائفة السنية تعتبر الطائفة الثانية من حيث الحجم ، أو قد تصبح كذلك قريبا .

ومن الواضح ان هذه التغييرات وما يتعلق بها من تغيرات ديموغرافية أخرى في تركيب

لقد توصل البحث الى نتيجة غير متوقعة، وهي أهمية الاختلافات القائمة بين الوسائل الشائعة لمنع الحمل ومدى استخدام تلك الوسائل لدى كل طائفة. ومما يبعث على الاستغراب ان الطوائف التي تتمثل فيها الصفات العصرية (كالكاثوليك وغير الكاثوليك من المسيحيين) قد شاع بينها استخدام الطرق التقليدية لمنع الحمل. كالسحب مثلا. في حين شاع بين الطوائف الأخرى سنية كانت أم شيعية طرق حديثة لمنع الحمل، كاستخدام الحبوب، كما ان الطوائف الأخيرة هذه كانت أكثر الماما بوسائل ربط الانابيب وغيرها من الاساليب المتطورة في هذا المجال. وقد كان الحد من تعليم الزوجة، وغير ذلك من مظاهر التأخر الاجتماعي عاملا على زيادة الاختلافات القائمة في هذا المجال بدلا من تقليص هذه الاختلافات كما كان متوقعا.

ولعل التعليل المعقول لما سبق الاشارة اليه، هو أن المسيحيين قد ساعدهم احتكاكهم الكبير بالفرنسيين، ونمط تنقلهم وهجرتهم من الغرب واليه على سبق السنة والشيعة في استخدام وسائل منع الحمل تلك الوسائل التي لم تكن متيسرة الا على شكل وسائل السحب والطرق التقليدية الأخرى. كما وان اعتماد المسيحيون عليها اعتمادا كبيرا جعل منها عادة شائعة بينهم في حين كان السنيون والشيعة الذين لم تتح لهم الفرصة استخدام الوسائل المذكورة مهيئين لاتباع طرق أخرى أكثر تطورا.

ومن خلال التحليل، تم أيضا التوصل الى مفهوم أساسي يمكن الاستفادة منه الى أبعد الحدود، يتمثل هذا المفهوم بأنه من الخطأ التعميم في تحديد سلوك الأفراد تجاه الخصوبة استنادا الى عقائدهم وتعاليمهم الدينية الرسمية. فغالبا ما يلاحظ خطأ البحاثة والمخططون الذين يعتمدون في دراستهم على تأثير الاسلام على الخصوبة، فيما يتوصلون اليه من قرارات. وهم بذلك أكثر خطأ من أولئك الذين يعتمدون على دراسة أثر المسيحية أو اليهودية على الخصوبة. فبينما دراسة الكتب الدينية وتفسيراتها تعتبر محاولة مجدية لفهم نشوء العقائد والعادات والاتجاهات الدينية. يلاحظ ان الاعتماد على ذلك في تفسير السلوك الحالي للخصوبة مضللا. فبدلا من الاعتماد على تفسير آيات القرآن الكريم والاحاديث النبوية الشريفة وغيرها من المفاهيم الدينية، يجب ان يعتمد علماء الاجتماع ورجال الدين المعنيون بتنظيم السياسة السكانية على تكييف الأحوال وفقا لكل طائفة بما يتلائم مع تطلعاتها الاجتماعية والاقتصادية، والوقوف على القوى المحركة لسلوكها الانجابي.

هناك نتيجة هامة أخرى، توصل اليها التحليل في هذا البحث، وخاصة، من خلال معالجته للواقع السائد في لبنان، ذلك البلد العربي المتعدد الأديان. تتلخص هذه النتيجة بأنه – وبغض النظر عن أية طائفة دينية معينة، وبعد التسليم بأثر الدين على الخصوبة والمواقف المختلفة تجاه تنظيم الاسرة، فان هناك عوامل هامة أخرى، كمجمل دخل الأسرة، ومركز رب الأسرة المهني وتعليم الزوجة، ومساحة المسكن ... ترتبط ارتباطا ايجابيا بعمليات تنظيم الأسرة ومعرفة استخدام وسائل منع الحمل. من هنا كان على أولئك المعنيين بالمعدلات السريعة للنمو السكاني في دول منطقة الشرق الأوسط أن يأخذوا هذه العوامل بالحسبان ويعتبروها مشجعة، اذ ان الارتقاء بالمستويات المعيشية للسكان وزيادة الرفاه الاجتماعي والاقتصادى، وبالتالي سهولة الحصول على

ان الفروق النهائية الهامة الخاصة بالخصوبة، والقائمة بين السنيين من جهة والمسيحيين الكاثوليك وغير الكاثوليك والدروز من جهة ثانية (والمتعلقة بالزوجات ذوات المستوى التعليمي المنخفض) كانت منسجمة مع المواقف تجاه عمليات تنظيم الأسرة ومعرفة وسائل منع الحمل واستخدامها. غير ان هذه الفروق لم تكن متطابقة مع الحجم المرغوب فيه للأسرة. فقد كانت الطائفة السنية متفقة مع غيرها من الطوائف الثلاث الاخرى فيما يتعلق بعدد الأطفال المرغوب فيهم، حيث كان هذا المعدل ٣ر٥ طفلا للدروز، و ٣ر٧ طفلا للمسيحيين غير الكاثوليك، ٣ر٩ طفلا للسنيين، و ٣ر٩ طفلا للكاثوليك. هذا، ولقد استمر ثبات هذه النتائج حتى بعد تحييد التغيرات الديموغرافية والاجتماعية والاقتصادية. ومع ذلك، برزت اختلافات واضحة في المواقف تجاه تنظيم الأسرة ومعرفة وسائل منع الحمل واستخدامها بين السنيين من جهة، والكاثوليك وغير الكاثوليك من المسيحيين وكذلك الدروز، من جهة ثانية. وقد كان هذا متوقفا أساسا على المستوى التعليمي الذى توصلت اليه الزوجة. ومن الزوجات الأميات ذوات المستوى التعليمي المنخفض كانت السنيات أقل الماما واستخداما لوسائل منع الحمل، كما كّن أيضا أقل تأييدا لتنظيم الأسرة من مثيلاتهن المسيحيات الكاثوليك وغير الكاثوليك وكذلك من الدروز، كما ان نسبة الخصوبة للنساء السنيات كانت أعلى مما هي لدى الطوائف الثلاث الأخرى. لقد اختلفت هذه الصورة تماما لدى النساء المتعلمات تعليما عاليا فقد بدت الاختلافات بسيطة بين السنيات وغيرهن من نساء الطوائف الثلاث الأخرى، فيما يتعلق بالمواقف الخاصة بتحديد النسل، وكذلك بمعرفة واستخدام وسائل منع الحمل. يضاف الى ذلك ان فروق الخصوبة بين النساء السنيات وغيرهن من هذه الطوائف كانت أيضا طفيفة للغاية.

أما فيما يختص باختلافات الخصوبة النهائية بين الكاثوليك وغير الكاثوليك من المسيحيين والدروز، فقد كانت ضئيلة سواء فيما يتعلق بحجم الأسرة الامثل، والمواقف المتخذة من تنظيم الأسرة والالمام بوسائل منع الحمل وممارستها. وقد تكون أبرز هذه الاختلافات البسيطة متركزة حول موضوع الحجم الأمثل للأسرة وتحديد هذا الحجم (وهو أمر لم تجر هذه الدراسة قياسا له) مثال ذلك شدة الاختلافات الدينية الخاصة بالتمسك بتحديد الحجم الأمثل للأسرة، أو مدة ممارسة وسائل منع الحمل.

ثمة نتيجة هامة برزت بجلاء أثناء المعالجات والتحليلات التي قامت بها هذه الدراسة، وتتمثل هذه النتيجة في أن المقارنات البسيطة التي عقدت بين الديانتين الاسلامية والمسيحية لم تكن ذات مدلول خاص. فقد وجدت اختلافات كبيرة وهامة فيما يتعلق بالخصوبة بين الطوائف المتعددة للديانة الواحدة. كما وجدت هذه الاختلافات بالنسبة لتحديد الحجم الأمثل للأسرة والمواقف الخاصة من تنظيم الأسرة والالمام بوسائل منع الحمل وممارستها. ففي حالات كثيرة كانت المعدلات والنسب تتشابه لدى الطوائف الاسلامية والمسيحية. كما أظهرت المقارنات، في بعض الأحيان، فروقا بين المذاهب الخاصة بالدين الواحد تتعدى تلك الفوارق الموجودة بين الديانتين المذكورتين، ان لم تفقها حجما. من هنا كان اعتماد سياسة مبنية على الاختلافات البسيطة القائمة بين الديانتين أمرا مضللا ان لم تؤخذ بالحسبان الاختلافات القائمة بين المذاهب الخاصة.

من هذا المنطلق، فقد كان التاريخ السياسي ونمط التحرك السكاني ، اضافة للانتماءات والروابط وغيرها من العوامل، من الامور المساعدة في تحديد سلوك المجتمعات الدينية المبحوثة نحو موضوع الخصوبة وتنظيم الأسرة، فموقف الفئتين المسيحيتين يعتقد بأنه أقل ايجابية للانجاب من موقف المسلمين، وبكلمة أخرى، فقد كانت نظرتهما لتنظيم الأسرة أكثر تأييدا منه لدى الطوائف المسلمة. وبالمقابل فقد كانت نظرة الدروز الى تنظيم الأسرة أكثر جدية منه لدى السنة والشيعة.

من جهة ثانية، فقد اهتم هذا البحث بمدى الاختلافات الديموغرافية والاجتماعية والاقتصادية السائدة بين الطوائف الدينية الخمس. والصورة التي برزت هنا تشير بوجه عام الى وجود اختلافات كبيرة في الابعاد الاجتماعية والاقتصادية بين الديانتين الكبيرتين، الاسلامية والمسيحية. كذلك برزت هذه الاختلافات بوضوح بين الطوائف المسلمة. وفي كل مقياس اجتماعي واقتصادى كان ترتيب المذاهب متشابها تقريبا من حيث الخصوبة وتنظيم الأسرة، حيث يأتي الكاثوليك من المسيحيين في القمة، يليهم الدروز ومن ثم السنة وأخيرا الطائفة الشيعية.

ومن الناحية التحليلية الأخرى، أى دون مراعاة الاختلافات الاجتماعية والاقتصادية، فقد برزت فروق كبيرة للخصوبة بين المذاهب الدينية المختلفة، مسيحية كانت أم اسلامية، بحيث يمكن ترتيب هذه المذاهب وفقا لارتفاع مستويات الخصوبة من الادنى الى الأعلى حسب ما يلي: غير الكاثوليك من المسيحيين يليهم الكاثوليك والدروز ومن ثم السنيون وأخيرا الشيعة.

لقد دعم تطبيق الافتراض التفاعلي على لبنان نتائج التحليلات السابقة التي استخلصها هذا البحث، فقد وجد، بعد تحييد الاختلافات الديموغرافية والاجتماعية الاقتصادية بين الطوائف الدينية، ان الفوارق في النسبة التجميعية للخصوبة تتوقف على المستوى التعليمي للمرأة. فعند المستوى التعليمي المنخفض بدت فوارق الخصوبة كبيرة، (لا سيما بين السينيين والشيعة) في حين أن هذه الفوارق لا تكاد تذكر عند المستويات التعليمية المتقدمة.

من جهة أخرى، بدت الفروق النهائية البارزة للخصوبة بين صفوف طائفة الشيعة وبين غيرها من الطوائف متطابقة مع الاختلاف في الحجم المرغوب فيه للأسرة، وكذلك مع المواقف المختلفة لتنظيم الأسرة والالمام بوسائل منع الحمل وممارسة هذه الوسائل. هذا، ورغم تحييد التغييرات الديموغرافية والاجتماعية والاقتصادية، فقد أعرب الشيعيون عن أعلى متوسط للعدد الأمثل للاطفال في الأسرة (٤ر٥ طفلا) كما أبدوا رغبتهم في انجاب اعداد أكبر من الأطفال في الأوضاع المناسبة. ومن الزوجات ذوات المستوى التعليمي المنخفض كانت النساء الشيعيات أقل تأييدا لتحديد النسل، كما كن أقل الماما بوسائل منع الحمل واستخداماتها. وقد توصل البحث الى أن الفروق الخاصة بالخصوبة كانت، عند هذا المستوى التعليمي المنخفض على أشدها بين الطائفة الشيعية والطوائف الدينية الأخرى. كما توصل البحث أيضا الى وجود ارتباط عكسي بين نسبة التعليم ونسب الالمام بوسائل تنظيم الأسرة واستخداماتها بين صفوف الطائفة الشيعية بحيث تتضاءل الفروق الدينية الخاصة بالخصوبة.

موجـــز البحـــث في اللغـــة العربيـــة

يتمثل الهدف الرئيسي من هذا البحث في تحديد طبيعة تأثير العقيدة الدينية على الخصوبة والعلاقات المتبادلة بينهما. لقد قاد قصور تطابق التفسيرات النظرية للاختلافات الدينية للخصوبة مع النتائج العملية للبحث الى اقتراح الافتراضات (دعيت بالافتراضات التفاعلية) تلك الافتراضات التي لم تنسجم مع النتائج التي توصلت اليها الابحاث المماثلة السابقة، فقط بل اضافت اطارا منهجيا لهذا البحث. وباختصار فان الافتراضات التفاعلية قد أكدت أن القيم الدينية وما تؤديه من توجيه خاص لدى محبذى الانجاب كان لها تأثير أساسي أثناء التحول الديموغرافي، ذلك ان هذا التأثير قد خفف من عوامل تكيّف لدى المؤمنين بهذه القيم، مع الظروف الجديدة التي تعتبر الخصوبة المنخفضة أمرا مناسبا. ويمكن القول بأن مستويات الخصوبة التي سبقت مرحلة التحول الديموغرافي كانت مقبولة من الجميع، بمعنى أن العوامل الدينية لم تكن ذات موضوع في تباينات الخصوبة. أما بعد مرحلة التحول الديموغرافي، فقد أدى تطوّر الاوضاع في المجتمعات الحديثة في النهاية الى الغاء دور أثر العقيدة الدينية على الخصوبة.

لقد اعتمد هذا البحث على البيانات التي وفرها المسح الذى نهضت به جمعية تنظيم الأسرة اللبنانية عام ١٩٧١ عن الخصوبة وتنظيم الأسرة على المستوى الوطني في لبنان. وقد شمل ذلك المسح عينة مقدارها ٢٧٩٥ من الأزواج وزوجاتهم. بشرط أن يتراوح عمر الزوجة بين ١٥–٤٩ سنة. ويكتسب هذا المسح أهمية ليس من منطلق تصوير نتائجه للاختلافات الدينية للخصوبة القائمة في لبنان فحسب، وانما أيضا من طبيعة الشعب اللبناني الذى لا توجد بين أفراده اختلافات عرقية أو عنصرية هامة.

وبالرغم من أن لبنان يضم حوالي ١٧ طائفة دينية، فان المسح الوطني للخصوبة وتنظيم الأسرة قد ميّز بين طوائف خمس فقط هي : من المسلمين (١) السنة (٢) الشيعة (٣) الدروز. أما من المسيحيين فقد ميّز (٤) الكاثوليك (غالبيتهم من الموارنة (٥) غير الكاثوليك (غالبيتهم من الروم الارثوذكس).

في المعالجات التي يتضمنها هذا البحث، سوف يتم التمييز بين الواقعين، واقع العقيدة الرسمي والواقع الفعلي للطوائف الدينية في لبنان، وذلك فيما يتعلق بموضوع الخصوبة وتنظيم الأسرة. ذلك لان الاعتماد على المذاهب الرسمية قد يؤدى بالنسبة لموضوع هذه الدراسة الى نوع من عدم الوضوح، وبصورة خاصة في مجال تحليل الاختلافات الدينية للخصوبة وتفسيرها. لذلك، فقد اعتمدت هذه الدراسة على معالجة الموضوع من زاوية التكيّف الذاتي للأسرة ضمن المجموعة الدينية الواحدة.

Index